P L A Y S

MARGUERITE YOURCENAR

~ ~

Plays

Translated from the French by Dori Katz
In Collaboration with the Author

Performing Arts Journal Publications
New York

Library of Congress Cataloging in Publication Data
PLAYS by Marguerite Yourcenar
Library of Congress Catalog Card No.: 83-62616
ISBN: 0-933826-63-X (cloth)
ISBN: 0-933826-64-8 (paper)

Design: Gautam Dasgupta
Printed in the United States of America

Publication of this book has been made possible in part by a grant from the National En-
dowment for the Arts, Washington, D.C., a federal agency, and public funds received
from the New York State Council on the Arts.

PAJ Playscripts/General Editors:
Bonnie Marranca and Gautam Dasgupta

Contents

Translator's Preface

Except for *Render Unto Caesar*, the plays in this collection were written in the forties when Marguerite Yourcenar had left Greece and France to visit the United States. *Electra or the Fall of the Masks* and *To Each His Minotaur* are taken from Greek legends; *The Little Mermaid* is based on the Hans Christian Andersen fairy tale. *Render unto Caesar* is inspired from her own previous work; the play is a dramatization of her novel *Denier du Rêve* (*A Coin in Nine Hands* in English).

As divergent as they first appear, all four plays concern the lack of fixed identities, the prevalence of illusion, uncertainties, self-deceptions, and betrayal. They are thematically related to the rest of Marguerite Yourcenar's writing.

Render unto Caesar was written in 1961. The plot is set in Rome in 1933 and revolves around a young, idealistic woman's attempted assassination of Mussolini. Before going off to her tragic fate, Marcella has three important confrontations: one with the wife of Carlo Stevo, her hero; one with her estranged husband whose political attitudes of collaboration with the regime she despises but whose body she still desires; and a final scene with a young accomplice she loves and who turns out to be a double agent. The dialogue offers attempts of justification and explanations for past and projected actions, and as such, the play is more psychological than political; its subjects are the cares, the preoccupations and routines of nine characters meeting in Rome.

As is the case in all of Marguerite Yourcenar's dramatic works, relationships are also problematic in *Render Unto Caesar*. Contemporary politics demand deception, half-truths, masks, illusions, borrowed poses, but the impossibility of objective truth is due more to personal reasons than to political ones. Deception is always self-deception, and "real" contact between characters occurs through luck rather than volition, and when it does occur, it is usually ignored, or noticed too late.

Electra or the Fall of the Masks was written in 1944 and is based on Euripides' *Electra*. In the modern play, Electra is married to Theodore, a peasant with whom she lives a wretched, difficult life of poverty in a miserable hovel. She has been sustained through all these difficult years of hardship by a burning thirst for revenge against her mother Clytemnestra and Aegisthus, her stepfather, and by her hope for Orestes, her brother, to return so that he will help her kill her enemies. The day he does return, she lures her mother to the house with the false rumor that she is pregnant and about to deliver her child. Once Clytemnestra arrives with a basket of food (not unlike Little Red Riding Hood going to visit Grandma and walking into the wolf's den) Electra kills her.

The moral fiber of the play changes when it is revealed that Aegisthus and not Agamemnon is Orestes' father. The news makes Orestes the son of a killer and not that of a victim. The weak, young Orestes is unable to change his mind; he carries out the murder, not caring anymore which of the two men is his father. The adulterous couple of Clytemnestra and Aegisthus are presented under a rather sympathetic light in their devotion to each other and their experience of life. The most admirable character of the play is Theodore, Electra's humble husband, who because of his sincerity, his unfaltering attachment to his wife, and his undeviating simplicity of purpose and feeling, forms a contrast to the ambiguous other characters.

To Each His Minotaur (1943) is an allegorical "divertissement sacré." It is a divertissement because it is mostly in a tone of light comedy or parody. It is sacred because it embodies ideas on life, death, good and evil; it can be compared to some other important writings of the author. It is based on Theseus' adventures in the labyrinth. The themes of the play are those of imposture and fatality, destiny and grace. Theseus fighting the minotaur is not dealing with a monster but is unknowingly confronting himself. The ghostly voices in the dark corridors are none other than those of memory and prophecy. Theseus does not recognize them and thus continues along his fatal path; he abandons Ariadne on an island after killing the minotaur (or did he?). In this context, Ariadne is an allegory for the soul. Bringing Phaedra home with him instead of his wife will lead to the violent death of Hippolytus, Theseus' son. Ariadne meets Bacchus, who is God, on the island where she is stranded; he leads her to death and salvation.

Certain scenes in this play cannot help but bring the agonies of historical victims to mind. The fourteen men and women plucked from their homes, transported to the inescapable labyrinth where they will be destroyed by an unknown monster, seem to evoke the deportees transported to concentration camps. They also recall the Africans abducted from their native lands and carried away in slave ships to the shores of America. While other such tragic connections can be made, in this play, the image of the ship sailing to Crete is, above all, that of mankind enclosed on the moving planet going towards in escapable death, and to what is God, for each of the passengers. Their reactions to their plight are as varied as the individuals, and they range from hedonism to anguish and fervor.

In this version of the legend, the nature of evil remains problematic; Theseus, after all, does not vanquish the monster. The human sacrifices end when the hero comes out of the labyrinth, but further death and tragedy wait, however, in the wings—the minotaur is still alive in other forms.

The Little Mermaid was written in 1942 while Marguerite Yourcenar was living in Hartford, Connecticut. Her friend Everett Austin, the brilliant art director of the Wadsworth Museum, a gifted amateur actor and theatrical director, was staging a show based on the four elements. He asked her to write something for "water"; this theatrical divertissement based on the fairy tale was the result. Of the four plays in this collection, it has the distinction of having been staged in the United States, in a since lost English translation by Grace Frick.

The play revives the story of the young mermaid who changes elements for the sake of love. The young creature must trade her beautiful voice for a pair of legs so that she can painfully walk on the hard ground behind her prince. As in the Andersen tale, here too the man does not recognize the true face of love and chooses to marry someone else. At the end of the play, the little mermaid leaves the deck of human beings and throws herself back into the sea, into the primordial world she came from.

1942 was the year that Marguerite Yourcenar became acquainted with Maine (where she still has a residence today), with a seacoast whose blue and gray landscape informs this play. It is the year her mind turned from meditation on mankind to meditation on land, from archeological concerns to, as she said in her preface to the 1970 French edition of this play, geological preoccupations—perhaps the little mermaid was the symbol and prefiguration of that change.

Dori Katz
October 1983

Render Unto Caesar

A Play in Three Acts

[1961]

List of characters in order of their appearance:

Lina Chiari
Paolo Farina
Clément Roux
Giovanna Stevo
Giuseppa Lovisi
Angiola Fides
Mother Dida
Maxime Iakovleff (Massimo)
Dr. Alessandro Sarte
Giulio Lovisi
Father Cicca
Rosalia di Credo
Marcella Ardeati
The Lady of the Cafe
The voice of the poet
The voice of the Dictator
Oreste Marinunzi

The following characters are walk-ons with a few lines:

A Fascist Guard (Tommaso)
Miss Jones
A few worshippers
A beggar
A theatre usher
A spectator
A high-ranking official

The following characters are walk-ons with no lines:

A newspaper vendor
A waiter
Some patients waiting for Dr. Sarte
A choirboy
A few spectators
An officer
A few guards
A driver

The play takes place in Rome, from April 20 to the 21st, 1933, in the Year XI of the Fascist Era.

ACT I

SCENE 1

An outdoor café. The light indicates broad daylight. At first, one sees only Paolo Farina and Lina Chiari seated at a table of the cafe. Lina is talking loudly, rapidly, complaining in an affected voice.

LINA: I am not saying that a hundred lira bill is not enough; I'm saying that it is not much. Naturally, you only come one day a week; the rest of the time, I manage as best I can to earn a living. But just the same, you breeze in from Pietrasanta every Monday and you stay till Tuesday, leaving by the 11:17 express. Regular as clockwork. It's not that I am complaining: you take me to the café; you treat me to a movie; when the weather is nice, off we go, you and me, for a little walk to Villa Borghese. Well, for me, it's as though it was a holiday, and how I manage the other six days, you couldn't care less. You're not that stingy with your sister-in-law.

PAOLO: Leave my sister-in-law out of this, Lina.

LINA: And how! That beanpole selling candles and holy virgins in plaster at Santa-Maria-Minore! Between the two of you, it's understandable that your wife split, without warning.

PAOLO: Leave my wife out of this, Lina. And lower your voice, people can hear.

LINA: What people? We're almost by ourselves. (*The light reveals, in turn, people seated at other tables: Clément Roux in front of a glass of beer; Giovanna and her mother, Giuseppa, with packages around them, drinking lemonade; a fascist guard in black shirt; a newspaper vendor. Lina barely glances at them.*) Hmm. You know, Paolo, people here don't stick their nose in their neighbor's business.

It's not like in Pietrasanta.

PAOLO: Leave me alone with Pietrasanta, my little Lina.

LINA: You seem upset. Am I teasing you too much? It's that I'm nervous, my big darling, very nervous. I'm losing weight, see. It looks good on me, right? But I had to take all my dresses in. And then, I don't sleep very well at night. Try to sleep late in the morning, the trucks going by to the market make such a noise . . . The other day I asked the pharmacist for a sedative. They don't grow on trees: fifteen lira! And no effect whatsoever, it's as though I swallowed pure water. Maybe I should go see a doctor. And last week, I had a sort of nightmare. A crab was stuck to my left breast. My flesh was blue, torn, crushed, bleeding. I screamed so loud I woke up the landlady.

PAOLO: That's enough, Lina.

LINA: (To herself.) He's like all the rest: if I'm sick or not, he doesn't give a damn. It's natural. He's not paying me to tell him my nightmares. And he didn't even notice this lump on the left side. All in all, it's a good sign: it's such a tiny lump. (To Paolo.) I don't want to bore you with my dreams, honey. But it really happened, that business with the crab. It was when I was still in the convent, when the sisters took the kids on an excursion to Bocca d'Arno. Because, you know, I'm sort of from the same place as you, which is why we get along so well, you and I. My father came from a little village around Pietrasanta.

PAOLO: I know, I know. You already told me all that, Lina. (To himself.) Angiola was also brought up in a convent in Florence, only it was a convent for noble women. Obviously, I wasn't the right husband for her. The daughter of a Sicilian Count isn't made to become Signora Farina. Even after what happened and the Marquis left her . . . I know that I have never been able to take care of their investments, since then, with the same devotion. All in all, I married her out of pity. No. No. You were in love with her, you wanted her. You still want her. But you will never see her again. You hired a private detective to find her; they really cheated you, those people, even though you are the financial director of the Princes of Trapani's affairs and the manager of their estates in Toscany. But no news, and no one has had any news in five years, and even Rosalia doesn't know anything. And she would rather die abroad, or enter a brothel than come back to your snug little home in Pietrasanta. If at least she had had that child of the Marquis, and he would have had your name (pater est quem nuptia demonstrant, of course), maybe she would have stuck around because of the kid. But no such luck. You'll never see your Angiola again, never . . .

(The light reveals Angiola Fides very elegantly dressed, walking by the café terrace. Paolo doesn't see her; his back is turned to her.)

LINA: (To herself.) What a beautiful hat! A French hat, a dress like the one in the last issue of *The Italian Woman*. And summer furs, the kind that aren't even useful! And I bet her underwear is the finest of the fine; not like you, though you still have to be all decked out to earn a living. A husband or a rich lover. Still, all in all, I'm glad to have Paolo every week with his hundred liras . . . He's a little stingy, like all serious clients . . . (*To Paolo.*) What are you thinking about, honey?

PAOLO: Nothing. I'll have another sandwich before catching my train. Waiter!

(*A waiter comes out of the shadows carrying a tray with a sandwich. Paolo pays, and counts his change very carefully, examining and turning over each coin.*)

LINA: Me, I'm interested in your Toscany, you know, honey. Daddy drove a carriage in Florence; his station was on Piazza Santa-Maria-Novella. And that's why, me, I know what they're thinking about, the coachmen with their carriages all lined up along the sidewalk, in front of cafés, like here, and how they worry when there aren't any tourists. Daddy had two horses; they were called Buono and Bello, and they were better treated than us kids. But Buono became sick and had to be put away. He had to be put away . . .

PAOLO: (*To himself.*) A little whore. The daughter of poor people raised, out of charity, in a convent in Florence. Not an institution for noble women like with my Angiola. And me, an upstanding citizen, a Party member, the manager of the estates of the Princes of Trapani in Toscany. I couldn't very well be seen in Pietrasanta with the likes of her. But this trip to Rome, every week, on the Prince's business, it's a little bit like going abroad. And it's true: when she talks, it's kind of like the other one, kind of the same voice, the same way of saying "Enough!" or "Let me sleep." I really should give her a little something, now and then, to make her happy.

(*Mother Dida comes out of the shadows and walks around the table with her flower baskets.*)

DIDA: Beautiful carnations, beautiful roses . . . Freshly cut, my beautiful roses . . .

LINA: Buy me flowers, honey. (*To herself.*) I shouldn't ask him that; it's not his style.

(*Paolo dismisses Dida automatically, by habit. Then:*)

PAOLO: Look. Lina, a brand new coin. With the fascist emblem, of course, and the date of the Year XI. Shiny like the beautiful silver coins from before the war. Here, I'm giving it to you. Wouldn't you like to have it? It's almost a good luck charm, see?

LINA: A little extra. Like a sort of tip? No, I was only kidding, honey: I'll put it with my four leaf clover. Next Monday? But, of course, but why not? I'll be here, naturally. Don't miss your train.

PAOLO: (*Leaving, accompanied by a spotlight.*) She's right when she says that here nobody looks at me; I'm this fellow sitting at a table with a whore. But in Pietrasanta, they know. An upstanding citizen. A member of the Party. The lawyer who, no matter what else they may say, won the case for the Mayor Tibaldi against that hydraulic company. The vice-president of the philately club . . . No, the fool who, one night, five years ago, found his house empty, and his wife gone with an actor, the husband cheated on, whom the neighbors pretend to pity. The cuckold . . . Angiola's cuckold. (*He disappears.*)

LINA: (*Left alone.*) Twelve after eleven. But on the clock there, it's already a quarter past eleven. When you're waiting, clocks and watches beat like hearts. Drink your cappucino slowly; pretend you're looking at your wristwatch, very obviously—first, because it's true, you want to know what time it is, then, so that the waiter really understands that you are here because you're waiting for someone. And not because you are too tired to get up and leave, and not either because you're trying to pick up a customer, like for example that old man, sitting at the next table, drinking. (*The light reveals Clément Roux for a moment. He's looking attentively at Lina.*) You don't really give a damn about the old man at the next table. Wait very quietly. God, make Massimo come! After all, it's your business to wait. You've probably spent more time waiting for customers than you have jacking them off. It is lucky that fat Paolo left. You wouldn't have wanted Massimo to come while he was eating his sandwich. Furthermore, he's so discreet, my little Massimo, he would have walked by pretending not to notice, and without even smiling. He'll come out of his German archeological library. He's taking some sort of course there. He will have his papers, his books; he'll put his long thin hands on the table, almost on yours. His life will be full of problems, worries, like always, of things you can't really understand completely. You'll feel better in trying to make him feel better. And if, by chance, he has some money (from time to time, it happens) he'll buy you a hat, or he'll take you to a concert, and you will go, even though you don't like classical music, but he'll say goodbye before the end because he will have met some friend. All in all, he doesn't seem to like women very much, too bad. God, make Massimo come! And he is still the only one you had the courage to tell that you were scared of that thing you don't understand, on your left breast, and maybe, he'll have the address of that doctor, like he promised. Darling . . . Darling . . .

(*The light reveals Massimo, looking as she described him. He sits down next to her.*)

MASSIMO: Are you feeling better? No, not much, right? You seem tired; you are worried. By the way, I brought you the address of the doctor.

LINA: I feel better when you're here.

MASSIMO: So, your big client left, did he? Are you free now? I made an appointment for you for this afternoon, at 3:30.

LINA: This afternoon? Right away? I'm not dressed to go . . .

MASSIMO: Are you scared?

LINA: Yes. (*Looking at the address.*) He is well known, eh? I saw his name in the newspapers. How much do you think he'll charge for his examination, this big doctor of yours?

MASSIMO: We'll work something out. For you, not much.

LINA: You know him? You know all the famous people.

MASSIMO: Through somebody. I mean, I have friends who know him. (*To the waiter.*) What I want? Nothing . . . Or, yes, a cappucino.

LINA: You're nervous this morning. I can tell by your voice. Do you have problems? New problems?

MASSIMO: Let's not talk about me, Lina. You'll go see Doctor Sarte, and then you'll know what's what. You can't let this thing keep eating you, and, if by chance, it's nothing . . .

LINA: Right, if it's nothing? After all, maybe I'm being ridiculous. It doesn't even hurt. All in all, maybe I should have consulted my old neighborhood doctor, the one who . . .

MASSIMO: Yes, but you owe him money.

LINA: It's not only that. He's seen me many times, you know. It would be as if he was examining me just out of habit. Mama used to say that sometimes it's useful to go pray in a different church. And I still haven't thanked you. After all, we haven't known each other that long, you and me; in a way, we aren't even very close. Oh no, I understand, I don't insist. Only, it's even nicer of you to be interested . . . (*She is ready to burst into tears.*) And I'm losing weight, you know, I'm losing too much weight; it doesn't look good on me. And I have no one. And when an idea haunts you, a sort of fear . . .

MASSIMO: I know.

LINA: For example, I have dreams at night. Last night, I dreamt about a crab biting me.

MASSIMO: Crabs don't bite, Lina.

LINA: Until I bled. It was hanging on to me. I couldn't stand it. I yelled.

MASSIMO: Easy, Lina, easy. If everyone started to tell their nightmares . . . (*He gets up.*) I have to go.

LINA: Already? What about tonight? Are we going to see each other as we always do at seven o'clock, at the cafe Piazza Balbo?

MASSIMO: No, I absolutely have to see someone.

LINA: It's because I'd like . . . I would really like to tell you what the doctor . . . After all, there aren't many people you can . . . They don't listen. They are all so selfish, darling. You are the only one who . . . You really can't?

MASSIMO: I'll call you. I have your number.

LINA: Yes, but the landlady is in a bad mood. You see, my rent is . . . And then, your name . . . She doesn't trust foreigners.

MASSIMO: I won't leave my name.

LINA: Yes, but there is also your accent, German or Russian, it's hard to tell. Me, I find your accent cute. And tonight, there is that film with Angiola Fides at the Mondo Theater. Don't you want to go?

MASSIMO: I already told you that I'm busy.

LINA: You see, I haven't yet told you this. It's difficult. But when you're there, I'm a different person. It's as though the weather was suddenly better. Are you going?

MASSIMO: I'm in a hurry today, Lina. No, don't worry, don't cry; it's so useless . . . Goodbye . . . (*He leaves quickly, followed by a spotlight. He stops in front of the newspaper vendor.*) You don't have the evening papers yet? (*He disappears.*)

LINA: He forgot to pay for his cappucino.

SCENE 2

The offices of Doctor Sarte. Stage right, in a bright and hard light, the examination room of Doctor Sarte. Stage left, dimly lit, the waiting room where people come in, sit down, get up to take a magazine, sit down again, without speaking to each other. Among them are Clément Roux, then Giovanna Stevo, brought in, in turn, by a silent receptionist. This will last throughout the scene. Doctor Sarte is sitting at his desk. When the curtain rises, he is on the telephone. Half-dressed, Lina is sitting across from him. Out of modesty, or because she is cold, she is holding, against her chest, the dress she took off to be examined.

DOCTOR SARTE: All right then: you will reserve a bed in the San-Bonaventura pavilion, for next Friday, the 23rd. CHI-A-RI, Lina. I'll tell her to come around two o'clock, not any earlier. Yes, as usual. The operating room around eight o'clock in the morning.

LINA: (*To herself.*) He's younger than I thought. Good looking man . . . But he probably only goes with women of the best class, the kind that one sees on the Via Veneto. (*To Doctor Sarte.*) Doctor . . .

DOCTOR SARTE: It's all set.

LINA: Doctor, does it really have to be Friday? Couldn't we wait a week? Especially since it doesn't even hurt . . .

DOCTOR SARTE: I thought I told you that every day that goes by decreases your chances. You have already waited too long.

LINA: But an operation, Doctor? Today, there are such strong medications, X-rays . . .

DOCTOR SARTE: Do you think I want to operate on you for my own pleasure? Listen, I explained what the problem was: you should be able to understand me. You have seen a fruit, a peach with a little spot on it. When you cut it, you sometimes notice that the spot is bigger than you thought. It has to be removed so that it won't contaminate the rest . . .

LINA: And then, if the operation is, as you say Doctor, a success, it means I'll wake up . . . with my left breast . . . Doctor, you are a man . . . Could you picture . . . You couldn't . . . How do you want someone in my profession . . . (*She bursts into tears.*) I'd rather go away . . . I'd rather die.

DOCTOR SARTE: Don't work yourself up, Signora Chiari. Maybe we'll find only a benign tumor. Don't be so quick to reorganize your future. (*To himself.*) Her future . . . Six months . . . A year . . . One never knows. That swelling of glands under the armpit . . . And then, there is probably metastasis on the side of the liver. (*To Lina who keeps on crying.*) You are undernourished; you say that you sleep badly since you started worrying about this lump. Do you have the prescription? Try to come to the hospital in the best shape possible.

LINA: So soon . . . Doctor, do you think next Tuesday . . .

DOCTOR SARTE: Do you have someone to get in touch with? Family? A friend? No? It's easier that way, believe me. Only, try to come rested. You can get dressed again. (*The telephone rings.*) Excuse me. (*Into the telephone.*) Yes . . . No, a patient. What? . . . It was to be expected. A man with tuberculosis in that kind of climate, with those conditions . . . Ah. (*To Lina.*) You can go now. (*She exits right.*) Beaten? Yes, I understand . . . I am not asking any questions . . . May I know what about that death bothers you? A retraction? You were able to make him retract? Not completely spontaneously, I would think? No, I haven't seen the evening papers yet. Of course . . . Of course . . . The news of his death will be broadcasted later . . . Naturally . . . Thank you for telling me about it. No, not exactly a friend: a friend from long ago. Yes, I know that you know, Tomasso. No, I'm not in direct contact with her, but indirectly, I follow her rather closely . . . (*With an involuntary touch of irony.*) And you too, I suppose. No, no one, especially not her . . . In any case, perhaps I'll see you tonight at the reception at Palazzo Balbo. (*To himself, sitting at his desk, thinking.*) Carlo Stevo's death . . . I am not particularly interested in Carlo Stevo's death. A big name in Italian literature as the *Corriere della Sera* will cautiously say tomorrow. I didn't even read all his books. But her, but Marcella . . . The story of his retraction is in the newspapers by now. She must already know it, the authorized version. And, for the rest, the little Iakovleff probably told her . . . No, maybe not. He's not too anxious to seem too well informed. Am I glad she is suffering? No. I'll have time to stop by the Via Fosca, before the reception at Palazzo Balbo. Compromising. This stone around my neck that she was for me, a rebel, a militant, the daughter of an adversary of the regime . . . She'll know soon enough. And besides, she is so hard: she'll never forgive him his retraction. Let her spit on her clay-footed hero, or, on better yet, cry over him in a catacomb.

(He presses a button. Clément Roux is led in. About seventy years old. He is both robust and haggard. His clothes are of good quality but neglected. He is wearing a soft hat that is dented. Maybe a cape.)

CLÉMENT ROUX: You were recommended to me, Doctor Sarte, after I had a little spell that . . . I'm in Rome for a few days . . . Where is my card? I'm sure I have a card . . . *(He goes through his pockets, finds a card and gives it to Doctor Sarte.)* The other day, at the Villa Medicis . . .

DOCTOR SARTE: Sit down, Monsieur Clément Roux. Now about that spell you mentioned . . .

SCENE 3

The street. When the curtain rises, Lina Chiari is crossing the stage from left to right. She is supposedly walking in the street, along the sidewalk, and every now and then, glances at shop windows out of habit. The light indicates it is late afternoon.

LINA: Wednesday, Thursday, Friday, Saturday . . . Where will you be Saturday, at four thirty in the afternoon? Dead? No, that's not the way it happens; one doesn't die that quickly. A bandaged thing, a butchered thing, a woman who no longer has quite the breasts of a woman . . . Don't think about it; you'll start crying again. Or screaming. And you won't be seeing Massimo tonight; he's not available, you won't be able to tell him . . . And you certainly can't go tell your landlady, because then, she'll want you to pay your rent right away. Who can you tell, then? This gentleman walking by? This lady between two children? How startled they would be if you stopped them to tell them . . . "Here, Ladies and Gentlemen, something like this will happen to you also one day . . ." Therefore, no doubt, it's a malignant tumor . . . Don't you have anyone to get in touch with? Not even a dog, Doctor . . . Just look: how pretty that creme satin brassiere in the shop window, and over there, those shoes with a silver buckle. On sale. But you don't have that far to walk anymore, my poor girl. As my mother would say, you'll always be able to make it as far as death . . . You are tired. Stop for a while before this newspaper stall; pretend you're reading the headlines. The illustrious writer Carlo Stevo retracts his odious slanders against the heads of the Party. I don't know who that is. Tonight, at nine o'clock, Piazza Balbo, big speech by the chief of State. Monsignor Maneggio's operation was a success . . . Don't worry; yours won't be in all the newspapers. Hmm, there it is,

Angiola Fides' new movie playing at the Theater Mondo, from two o'clock on. But Massimo is not interested in that film. Tonight, you'll go to bed with your sedatives, try to sleep. Dying is not so difficult; one goes to God. You'll have to buy one or two white nightgowns; you can't very well be decently buried in your black lace . . . It would have been harder if Massimo had loved you. And it would be a good idea to send fat Paolo a postcard, since you won't be there Monday; one has to be polite with people. But you won't die. You'll change professions; you know how to sew. Of course, one starves doing that for a living. Or you could sell flowers, like Dida. Don't cry, my poor girl; it's so useless. Look at yourself in this shop window. Do you feel like living with a face like that? A haggard face; a gray complexion, rather yellowish . . . Colorless lips . . . Where is my lipstick? No, not here. Not here either. I must have left it at the doctor's. No, I'm not going to go back, take the elevator, speak to that sort of receptionist in a white smock. Luckily, there's the perfume-shop where Estella always buys her things, the one with the little old man . . . (*To Giulio Lovisi who suddenly appears above his counter.*) A lipstick, please.

LOVISI: What shade?

LINA: Strawberry, no, raspberry.

LOVISI: Coty?

LINA: Too expensive.

LOVISI: Of course, of course. Besides, all Italian brands are the best in the world. But all the same, look at this case: what a jewel, and for only five more liras.

LINA: All right. Coty. It doesn't matter. I'll put it in my purse. (*He gives her back her change.*) Thank you, Signor. (*Alone.*) And now, take your pocket mirror, and make your face up again into a proper face, the face of someone who is not sick and who has not been crying. First, powder. And then lipstick, and open your lips a little so you won't have a pale line at the corner of your mouth, and put a lot on so that it will be as red as a heart. Estella is always saying that there are three ways to hook men: first you walk slowly, turning around now and then, to show that you are available. Then you wear a dress that clings, and that shows your body, shows the form of the breasts (no, don't think about it, don't think about it anymore); and then, especially, lots of lipstick. Because, what they really like, are for women to be easy; they're such cowards, all of them. Now, with your fingertips, smear a little of your lipstick on your cheekbones; it's almost like real rouge; it makes you look feverish but pretty. How strange it is that it takes so little to look pretty . . . It's a shame that Massimo never gave me his telephone number. But there aren't that many places he could be at this time of day: maybe he's at the Bar Rosario. And if you run into him, he'll buy you an ice cream, or tomorrow you'll have dinner together in Monte-Mario, and you'll wear your dress with the pink stripes . . . Smile, my poor girl, you're prettier when you smile than when you cry. And furthermore, the doctor said it: one never knows . . . Maybe it will only be a tiny little scar. (*She disappears.*)

(*Allesandro Sarte coming out of his building appears, going straight towards the footlights. He is wearing a black raincoat over his evening clothes, and a white scarf.*)

DOCTOR SARTE: Don't take the car; useless and cumbersome on an evening when the streets are barricaded. I have all the time I need to have a quiet dinner at Rainier's and then walk to Palazzo Balbo. What a chore! And the other day, it was for the Nazi delegation: General Goering with all his rings . . . But on an evening like tonight, it's better to at least put in an appearance in the official circles. Tomasso will probably have some details to give me . . . And furthermore, even if one is well considered, approved, with the right passwords, Marcella's husband is still a man watched . . . Or at least, a man to watch . . . And if I go to Via Fosca tonight, it would be better that some over-zealous policeman does not take down the license number of my car parked at the door. Call a taxi. But I won't go on Via Fosca. I haven't resisted the desire to see her for months to run into a meeting of suspicious characters in a back room. "Absurd marriage!" as my father used to say. But a marriage, nevertheless, since I can no more forget this woman than I can my name, or the number on my identity card. Don't try to fool yourself; I will go to Via Fosca. Not that my decision not to go will weaken in the least, on the contrary. But I know that I will go, and I also know that it will be useless, ridiculous, and slightly indecent. I keep on walking in the opposite direction; I keep on going towards Rainier's; I keep on saying no, but the time will come (and I know it) when I'll say to the taxi driver, "Via Fosca." Strange mechanism. Everything happens as if there were in us different faculties of will.

SCENE 4

The church of Santa-Maria-Minore. As the curtain rises, the stage first shows a classical portal, placed on a slant on the left which is supposed to go from the street to the church. Mother Dida is sitting on the steps of the church between two baskets of flowers. Father Cicca, priest of Santa-Maria-Minore, comes in, hurrying to be on time for the evening benediction. The scene is lit by a bit of remaining sunset.

FATHER CICCA: (*Stopping for a moment on the threshold.*) Have a heart, Mother Dida! Give me a rose for the Holy Virgin!
DIDA: Not on my life! She's richer than me, your Holy Virgin!

(*Father Cicca sighs and goes inside the church where the heavily gilded altar lights up.*

In the nave, a small group of worshippers can be seen, either standing or sitting on chairs. Among them are Clément Roux, Miss Jones, Giulio Lovisi. In the foreground, on the right of the stage, is the stall of Rosalia di Credo with its candles, its little plaster virgins and its rosaries. The following conversation is spoken in whispers.)

ROSALIA: There you are, Signor Lovisi. And how is the dear little girl today?

LOVISI: A little better. Or rather no, about the same, Signorina di Credo, but one always says "a little better," you know, out of habit. With a father who has tuberculosis, you understand. And the new doctor says the same thing as the others, it will take time and endless treatments. It's hard, especially on her poor mother. (*To himself.*) On the contrary, it's rather lucky for my Vanna to have her child to worry about. She couldn't very well spend the whole day waiting for news of a prisoner.

ROSALIA: Poor angel! (*She lowers her voice.*) What a misfortune for your daughter that he didn't leave in time for Lausanne!

LOVISI: The fool. I always thought that man would come to a bad end. How many times did I tell him that, good God! No, I exaggerate, Signorina di Credo, I never would have had the courage to say anything. A famous man, while me, I didn't even finish elementary school . . .

ROSALIA: That doesn't keep you from knowing a lot about life, Signor Lovisi.

LOVISI: When I think that everything started because my wife wanted to live in Ostia, on account of her asthma, you know. By the seashore . . . And it isn't so practical for me with a store in town. Well, when we had to take a boarder, and when this well known writer came, looking for a quiet place to work, and fresh air to get over his pneumonia, how do you expect a passionate heart like my Vanna's, not to . . . Me, I could never bear that man.

ROSALIA: (*To herself.*) And me, I always disliked Paolo. It's wrong to dislike your brother-in-law. Still, he couldn't keep our Angiola.

(*Wordless scene: a choir boy walks around lighting lamps.*)

LOVISI: I'm exaggerating, Signorina di Credo, I'm exaggerating. I didn't dislike him yet at that time, no one knew that he was a criminal; he hadn't yet been condemned. And I was rather proud, when Vanna settled with him in a fine apartment in town. I had even accepted not to see her too often; they had better things to do than to invite me and Giuseppa. But writers, you know. One never knows what to expect. When Giovanna came back to us with her little girl, we realized that it is always a mistake to marry above your station. And even then, I didn't think that Vanna was completely in the right: she is difficult, like her mother.

ROSALIA: That's because it's difficult to be a woman, Signor Lovisi.

LOVISI: And things are not getting better, you know. He's in prison, we should all be living in peace now. Well, no, it's as if there was a ghost in the house.

ROSALIA: But what about him, Signor Lovisi, the poor man . . . Did they tell you . . . where he was?

LOVISI: Yes, on an island . . . I don't know which one . . . near Sicily.

ROSALIA: (*To herself.*) I was born in Sicily. And the house was Gemara, the only house in the world . . . And our father was not yet this poor old man that had to be put in an asylum. Angiola used to bathe in the sea, and when I called her, she would come bouncing like a little goat . . .

LOVISI: It wouldn't be so bad if our Vanna were a bit more reasonable. My wife has to get up in the middle of the night to pray with her, make her drink some warm milk, tuck her into bed again, well, you know, calm her. And all this because this Signor meddled in politics and is wiling away his time on a rocky island. And to think that it's always the innocent who pay! We can't sleep anymore.

ROSALIA: Patience, Signor Lovisi, patience!

(*Wordless scene. Miss Jones buys a candle from Rosalia.*)

LOVISI: Just think; having a son-in-law who dared attack such a great man! Our Great Man. And a man who succeeds in everything. When I think that we thought we were giving our Vanna to an educated man . . .

(*The organ starts a Bach fugue.*)

CLÉMENT ROUX: (*Sitting, to himself.*) Hmm, I was sitting peacefully on my chair, and all of a sudden, this noise breaking in . . . This noise, no it's the organ. But so suddenly that one didn't expect it. That's it: a second chord explains the first one, like in my painting, a second stroke of color next to the first. They seem like questions followed by answers, but these questions have a meaning and these answers also; it's not like in the world where we live. Yes the organ moves you, yet you never go to hear it at Saint-Germain-des-Prés or at Saint-Sulpice. No time . . . But here, in this gold coffer . . . So soft, their golds . . . But all in all, no one understands this music, not even me. Except perhaps the organist up there, but no matter what, you can feel its beauty. It even covers up the noise of the buses and taxis that irritated me a while back before this Bach fugue started. They seem used to their awful din, but me, it spoils Rome for me. I wonder if I did the right thing coming here for the opening of my show, at my age. There is not much time left; I still have things to finish in my studio. But what a shame that it's too dark to see that Caravaggio fresco again: in the chapel, on the right, the one that shows that seductive girl with a handsome young man wearing a feathered hat, so much more important, the two of them, than poor old Saint Peter. Well, still, I was right to come to Rome.

MISS JONES: (*Lighting her candle.*) I was right to buy this candle, even though the pastor in Putney would be very surprised . . . But since I have more change than I'll need before I leave Rome . . . Lord, make them give me a raise; make them make me secretary to the assistant-director; have the crossing tomorrow be calm . . . Even in a Catholic church, it always feels good to pray.

FATHER CICCA: Mother of God . . .

THE WORSHIPPERS: Pray for us . . .

FATHER CICCA: Endearing Mother . . .

THE WORSHIPPERS: Pray for us . . .

LOVISI: (*Sitting, to himself.*) It means a lot to me this little evening benediction at Santa-Maria-Minore, every night, before catching the 23 tram, and then the train at Porto-San-Paolo station . . . (Mustn't forget the package of ribbons under the chair; otherwise, there will be a scene!) The fact is, I'm not in such a hurry to go home to them, the grumbling mother and the daughter weeping or trying her best not to weep. My poor Giovanna! And the little one (I adore her!) is sometimes moody. But here, I am all right. The good Lord doesn't even ask that you pay a lot of attention to the prayers. She's not bad, that blonde in her travelling clothes, the English girl who doesn't know how to go about lighting a candle. So young . . . I bet she doesn't know much about love . . . A Protestant . . . Not even made-up, poor thing . . . I am a decent man, after all, others would do worse than going to evening benediction every night . . . And here, at least, Giuseppa isn't going to come to make a scene.

FATHER CICCA: House of gold.

THE WORSHIPPERS: Pray for us . . .

ROSALIA: (*To herself.*) A house, a house in Sicily. It's no longer ours; it's for sale. It will be sold to pay father's debts. They probably stuck an announcement that's getting crumpled and blown in by the wind, on the door, with the name of the real-estate agent in small black letters. The only house in the world, an old house, the house in Sicily . . .

FATHER CICCA: Queen of Angels . . .

THE WORSHIPPERS: Pray for us . . .

FATHER CICCA: Queen of Martyrs . . .

THE WORSHIPPERS: Pray for us . . .

MARCELLA: (*Coming in.*) Luckily I have my shawl, otherwise I couldn't have ducked into the church to get out of this downpour. This absurd superstition that won't let bare-headed women enter a church! And what's more, the folds of the shawl hide this package, this thing . . . Newly oiled . . . Hopefully the dampness won't hurt it. In any case, nothing to fear from the gun seller; he's a member of the Group. Sometimes, things work out. More often than you'd think, when you're determined to see it through to the finish, and not leave a way out behind you. It's a good thing that Alessandro taught me how to shoot in Reggiomonte . . . The balcony or the door?

In front of the balcony, in the crowd, it's harder to raise your arm. But they watch the door more. It is better, in the long run, that there be an alternative; you'll choose once you're there. Still, it might have been wiser to opt for the Villa Borghese . . . To manage to be near the horses' path; to look like a woman strolling with a child . . . No, no, don't hesitate . . . Soon, I will be dead, that is the only thing that is sure. What are they saying? Queen of the Heavens; *Regina Coeli*, this name of a prison! Is it there that tomorrow . . . See to it, please God, that I die right away. See to it that my death not be useless, that my hand not tremble, that he be killed . . . Well, how strange . . . Here I am, starting to pray without realizing . . .

FATHER CICCA: Ivory Tower.

THE WORSHIPPERS: Pray for us. . .

CLÉMENT ROUX: (*To himself.*) How beautiful these words are! Ivory tower. Even though the thought of it disgusts me, ivory, these beautiful great animals slaughtered. But me, (is it sacrilegious?) ivory makes me think rather of bodies. For example, that little girl on the beach, one evening, could it be already twenty years ago? I *am* tired: this stormy weather . . . let's hope that the new medication Doctor Sarte gave me . . . This woman wearing a shawl is beautiful: a simple beauty, without shadings, vigorous, in the classic style. I would be wise to sit here another few minutes, then I'll walk back to the hotel . . .

FATHER CICCA: Refuge of sinners. Health of the sick . . .

THE WORSHIPPERS: Pray for us . . . Pray for us . . .

ROSALIA: (*Leaning toward Giulio Lovisi, above her stall.*) You have your troubles, Signor Lovisi, with that sick little girl. Perhaps if you offered a candle to the Holy Mother . . . She is so kind!

LOVISI: (*Hesitating.*) Maybe, Signorina di Credo, maybe. A candle . . . (*To himself.*) A candle . . . No, two: Mimi, Vanna, and one of Giuseppa, to ask, dear God, that she leave me alone, and for Carlo, after all . . . We can't really hope that he will come back; this man would always be a suspect in the eyes of the authorities. But one has to be kind; one can, nevertheless, pray that his life not be so hard; it must not be much fun being a prisoner on an island. Four candles, Signorina di Credo, four candles. (*He rises.*)

ROSALIA: You're spoiling the Madonna, Signor Lovisi. What size?

LOVISI: Medium, Signorina. (*He lights the candles.*)

FATHER CICCA: Pray for us, poor sinners . . .

THE WORSHIPPERS: Now, and at the hour of our death . . .

LOVISI: We're all sinners, after all, Signorina Rosalia.

ROSALIA: (*Giving him back his change.*) We all do our best, Signor Lovisi.

THE WORSHIPPERS: SOBEIT . . . SOBEIT . . . SOBEIT . . .

MARCELLA: Words with no meaning, a sort of inept incantation, a magic formula . . . They don't even know anymore what they are saying. The opium of the poor: Carlo was right. They have been taught that all power comes from above. None of these people would be capable of doing what I'm going to do. None of these people would be able to stand up and say no.

(*The light on the altar goes out. One by one the worshippers leave.*)

SCENE 5

In a street lined with buildings. The portal of Santa-Maria-Minore still placed on the left of the stage is now seen from the front. A little further on, on the same side, a low house with an exterior staircase where Father Cicca lives on the second floor. On stage right, at an angle, the corner of the building where Marcella occupies the ground floor, and Rosalia, the fourth floor. Originating from a sort of interior courtyard, a staircase is buttressed against the building. The light is that of late twilight. Father Cicca and Rosalia di Credo greet each other on the Church porch as the curtain rises.

FATHER CICCA: A lovely evening. And a very good evening to you, Signorina di Credo.

ROSALIA: A bit stormy, though. Good evening, Father Cicca.

(*Father Cicca watches her walk off for a moment, then goes into the church, sighing. Rosalia crosses the stage, then slowly climbs the staircase on the right. The light follows her during her climb to her fourth floor apartment.*)

ROSALIA: (*To herself.*) And now your day is over. You have worked; you are going home. It's a very correct kind of job, a job that doesn't dirty your hands; a job suitable for a signorina of a good family who has seen better days . . . You are going home. Home? The house that is your home has probably been sold already, if only they found some buyers. Last Sunday, I went to the asylum to speak to Father. He didn't understand. Or he made believe he didn't understand. He doesn't want to understand that the house was sold to cover the unpaid debts; he doesn't want to know that our Angiola married badly, that she ran away, and that it's already been four years since anyone has heard . . . He was looking at me, and he was stroking the arms of the Asylum's wicker chair, and for him it was the mahogany armchair he left in Gemara. It's as though he managed to hold on to a place that they can't take away from him, and to daughters who haven't turned out wrong. His madness, it's his Sicily. And what about your Sicily, where is that? Go up the staircase. You will go up at night, and you will go down in the morning, every day of your life. And you're only thirty years old, and you're from a family where the women live a long time. And you will reach the top, slightly out of breath, and you will turn the key, and you will only find an empty room. And it will always be the same sounds, the same smells;

not a house for someone from a good family. Admit that you are rather pleased the old man left, that you no longer have to wash his sheets, get him something to eat. But the loneliness . . . At least, when we moved in here, Angiola was still at school; she would come back during holidays; you made her dresses; you would kneel before her, your mouth full of straight pins; you took care of her when she was in trouble. You even put up with that ridiculous husband she took because of the scandal. And now, you are alone. And you will remain alone. You didn't even get to know love; you have only had your father and your Angiola. Close the window; you won't hear the radio from across the way. Your soup . . . Where is the charcoal? No, you're out of it; your supper, you won't be able to heat it up. Ah, silly woman that you are, charcoal can be used for other things besides warming up your supper: it can be used for . . . You sit right next to the lovely embers; you lean over as if to smell the fiery flowers. You cough a little, but because you fall asleep, you don't notice that you're coughing. Ma-da-ma Cel-la! (*She leans out the window, calling Marcella down below, whom the light shows in what should be the courtyard of her back-shop.*)

MARCELLA: (*Startled, lifting her head.*) Who is it? You scared me. What can I do for you, Signorina Rosalia?

(*Rosalia lowers a basket with a long rope.*)

ROSALIA: Only a little bit of charcoal, Madama Cella. I put the money in the basket.

MARCELLA: Just a minute. (*She goes into the building.*)

ROSALIA: (*From above, dreaming, while Marcella who reappeared, puts the pan full of charcoal in the basket.*) You will not go down the stairs again; you won't go sell your rosaries, your candles and your little statues in plaster anymore. You will not end up like your father, in an asylum. You'll shut the window real tight, you'll block the cracks with a blanket. And you pull, you haul, like in the old days when you used to buy fruits or sweets for your Angiola from street vendors. And I'm pulling, and I'm heaving, and I'm hauling this charcoal, my death.

MARCELLA: Anything else?

ROSALIA: Nothing for the time being, Madama Cella.

MARCELLA: Just a minute, I'll go get your change.

ROSALIA: Later, Madama Cella. Good night.

MARCELLA: Good night, Signorina Rosalia.

(*The basket goes up. The light goes out. Father Cicca can be seen, under the portal of Santa-Maria-Minore, locking the church door. Then he leans over Dida, who is still sitting on the steps of the threshold. He speaks to her in a very loud voice because she is deaf.*)

FATHER CICCA: Dida! Hey, Dida! Do you hear me? She is deaf like those who don't want to hear. Your daughter, Marinunzi's wife, put her name down on the list of the poor of the parish. It's not surprising with four children, and a fifth one the good Lord is sending her. But you have money, mother Dida. You wouldn't need to sell flowers on the steps of Santa-Maria-Minore, if it wasn't that you like the work, and that you would be bored staying home in Ponte-Porzio. Everyone knows that there are beautiful brand new bills in the bag hanging around your neck like a scapulary.

DIDA: Enough, Priest! Those who talk like that will be to blame when Marinunzi cuts my throat some evening at the corner of a road. I am not about to milk myself dry for this scum who drinks up everything he gets. Work doesn't scare him; he sleeps right next to it.

FATHER CICCA: You're hard, mother Dida; no one ever saw you throw a dog a bone. You never slipped me a coin to say a mass for your good dead, and your two daughters, Tullia and Maria, the ones who are not quite right in the head, work like mules for you in your field in Ponte-Porzio. You will go to hell like all misers; you will be resurrected, hand clenched in a fist, and you will spend eternity trying, in vain, to open your hand again. Just think, Dida, an eternal cramp! But money that you give goes straight to the good Lord's savings account.

DIDA: And will the good Lord take care of me when my children have eaten up all my money, hey, little priest? (*To a beggar coming out of the shadows.*) Get out of here with your crutches! At this time of the day, the steps are mine alone.

(*She disappears in the darkness in the middle of a savage din of quarrel. Father Cicca turns left and slowly climbs the stairs of his building to the second floor.*)

FATHER CICCA: A little while ago, I couldn't find the right words to say to Signorina di Credo, who has family problems; and now, Dida, why did I need to quote Dante to her? You don't know how to speak to your parishioners, Father Cicca. You are the one who pronounces eternal words, and when they expect from you a simple word for them alone, you stutter. Everyone in the seminary always thought that you weren't very gifted. And meanwhile, they fret, they toss and turn, they suffer. You have been granted this terrible grace of being able to guess their wishes, their desires, their prayers; it's not always very pretty. "Me, me, me! . . ." They scream themselves hoarse. There are also those whom you do not understand very well; those who are marked by death, or those who are going to commit a crime . . . And you, you who judge them? You who pray to avoid another scolding by the bishop; you, who are jealous of your cousin who is in the insurance business and has a pretty little yellow car and a gold watch . . . You are not even very clean: look at the stains on your cassock. And you go back up into your sparse room, and you feel incompetent, useless. And, all of a sudden, the walls fly away: a flood of sweetness, like the purest of honey, flows in you; a breeze lifts you, a breeze fresher than any breeze of this world: these beautiful spaces, these beautiful stark spaces . . . God . . . God . . . God . . . How will you explain him, your God, to Dida who loves only money; how will you show him to that man who has you say a mass, from time to time, for a sick child; how will you assure Rosalia di Credo that God is everywhere and not only in a house in Sicily? How will you make them slide from the word *me* to the word *God*? And then, there is everything that is beyond your understanding; everything no one asks your opinion about: the government, the laws, the old ones and the new ones, the weak and the strong, the prisoners, the speeches of the chief of State. And sometimes you say to yourself that people render unto Caesar more than what belongs to Caesar. But don't mix everything up; those are not your priest ideas; they are your very own ideas, little Cicca. How will you go from all that to God? And that you be stupid is not what matters. Ah, Lord, why did you give me this certitude that is not granted others, this joy that I don't know how to share with them? As long as there will be, in the street, an old deaf woman, a blind beggar; as long as there will be a donkey bleeding under his pack, a starving dog roaming about, have me not fall asleep in the sweetness of God.

ACT II

Throughout this act, the set will consist of two rooms, center stage, which are Marcella's apartment. The room on the right, the first to be lit, has an entrance opening directly onto the Via Fosca. The room to the left will be seen only afterwards, when the light in the other room goes out. They are connected by a door. The rest of the stage remains dark and should be thought of as representing Via Fosca and other streets in this part of Rome. Shining through here and there, at different heights, lights must create the impression of windows and of street lamps in growing darkness.

SCENE 1

Marcella's room. Massimo and Giovanna are seen standing in the foreground, to the right, in what is supposed to be the threshold of Marcella's apartment. The whole scene is lit by a dim twilight light.

MASSIMO: This way. I'll go call her.

GIOVANNA: You see, I'm in a hurry. Since I live in Ostia . . .

MASSIMO: Come in. The hallway is no place to talk. And people walking by can hear. (*They take a few steps towards stage center.*) It's really almost night. Let me get some light.

(*The light shows just enough to suggest the inside of a room. A round table, some straw chairs. A coffee pot, two cups, a newspaper on the table that is well lit by an overhanging bulb. In the back, at the shadows' edge, a brass bed with a nightlamp shining on a religious print hanging slightly crooked. A chest of drawers with a wash basin and a pitcher.*)

MASSIMO: (*To himself, looking at Giovanna.*) So, it's her . . . Just about as he described her to me in Vienna. Bossy . . . Yet, timid. Dressed in black from top to bottom. In full mourning? No . . . Not yet. And furthermore if that were the case, she would already be wearing crepe from head to toe. Simply, a little bourgeois woman who thinks that black is always right.

MARCELLA'S VOICE: (*From offstage left, from where one can imagine a small court-yard off the back room. She is speaking to Massimo, dreamingly.*) Do you realize Massimo, that these pigeons ate all the seeds I put out for them just now? They walk on my hands . . . They take grains from my lips. And what strength in their little pink claws. But you know, I don't really matter. If by chance instead of me, a neighbor were to . . . tomorrow . . .

MASSIMO: (*Impatient.*) Come, Marcella, we are waiting for you here.

MARCELLA: (*Coming closer, half visible in the darkness that still submerges the room to the left.*) My little pigeon, why did you turn on the lamp? I have so many things to tell you tonight. It's better in the dark.

GIOVANNA: (*To herself.*) They're lovers? How shameful. And it's among these people that Carlo . . . What am I doing here with these shady characters, following this young man inside the house, like an accomplice . . . ?

MASSIMO: (*To himself, looking again at Giovanna.*) She has not read the evening papers either. Otherwise, she would be joyful, triumphant . . . As for Marcella . . . I am ashamed to be the only one who already knows.

(*Marcella, surprised but not disconcerted by the presence of the visitor, stops on the threshold of the fully lit room.*)

MASSIMO: Signora Carlo Stevo has come to ask us for news, Marcella.

GIOVANNA: (*Alarmed.*) He knows my name?

MARCELLA: (*Very heatedly.*) But I don't have any news! Tell her, Massimo!

GIOVANNA: (*Pushing Massimo back.*) Signora Marcella is the one I came to see.

MARCELLA: (*Firmly.*) Massimo Iakovleff wouldn't be here if he weren't up to date about everything. He was . . . He is . . . Signor Stevo's . . . best friend.

GIOVANNA: (*In an insulting way.*) I didn't expect you to refer to my husband so ceremoniously.

MARCELLA: (*Softly.*) Of Carlo then . . . our Carlo (*Even more softly.*) the poor man!

MASSIMO: Sit down, Signora Stevo.

(*They sit down. The three faces lit by the lamp are frozen for a moment in personal meditation. Giovanna is taking off her gloves, then mechanically unbuttoning her coat.*)

MASSIMO: (*He lights up a cigarette, also mechanically. To himself.*) Carlo Stevo . . .

Carlo Stevo . . . In spite of ourselves, we are talking about him as though he were dead. Here we are, the three of us, sitting around this table, as if holding a seance, and each of us conjures his own absent ghost. Carlo Stevo, a refugee in Vienna; that stranger in his threadbare clothes to whom a young man offered a false visa on a false passport; his faith, his terrible faith; and that strange sincerity that killed lies, my lies; and that fervor; and that passionate need for a disciple . . . What are you going to do with that memory the rest of your life?

MARCELLA: (*To herself.*) Carlo Stevo . . . Carlo Stevo's wife. Already married, I think, when Alessandro introduced him to me; he gave me Carlo, as he gave me so much else . . . it's only when I wanted to become independent again, free to come and go, useful, that I found this sort of hiding-place . . . It was a hiding-place for him too. From them? No, that would have been childish. But from her; from what she stood for. And when he came back from his voluntary exile, when I convinced him to act . . . This trip to Geneva when sympathizers helped us cross the border, those pamphlets slipped under doors in the wee hours of the morning, that despair that overwhelmed us both, as, sitting side by side in this room, we listened to the Dictator's voice thundering on the radio, that anguish that kept us awake all night long, the day before . . . Close to each other . . . I am right to try to do something tonight.

GIOVANNA: (*To herself.*) Carlo Stevo . . . And the future seemed sure. Success was right there; money was coming in, honors . . . The good life . . . Naturally, there was always the sadness because of the child. No, he really didn't want that kind of life; we were never quite enough for him. Those long absences; those dangerous acquaintances . . . Everything I never really understood . . . And yet, without this woman . . . He wasn't born to get involved in politics. Ah! Force yourself; speak to her anyway; try not to have come for nothing; manage to find out something. (*To Marcella.*) I have been without news now for three months. I am not in the habit of visiting strangers . . . But I thought . . . I told myself that perhaps you had connections we didn't have . . .

MARCELLA: Carlo writes to no one. We don't have any special connections, as you say, and as for official cards stamped by the governor of the island, if they contained anything that was essential, they would be intercepted. I don't see Carlo writing to say that the weather is nice and that he is feeling fine.

GIOVANNA: (*Misunderstanding, in a pompous way.*) But he is not feeling fine! Don't you remember that he sometimes spits up blood? Everyone thought he was cured, and then . . . Even when I was around to take care of him . . . Who knows if at the very moment I am speaking, the poor man is not dying in the prison hospital infirmary?

MARCELLA: Sick or not, as far as they're concerned it's all the same. You don't imagine that they will send him back to us alive?

GIOVANNA: And why not? A petition has been going around abroad. Everyone is counting on His generosity, on His clemency. People have been speaking of a, how do you call it, amnesty.

MARCELLA: Oh yes, I am well acquainted, at my cost, with his generosity and his clemency. My father was a friend in his youth when he was still only a militant socialist. My father supported him during some very hard times. And yet, he died destitute, dismissed from his wretched little job as a school teacher, scoffed at, slandered . . . And I almost lost my job as a nurse. Do you believe in the tirades in the newspapers, in the assurances that order and justice reign supreme even in the island barracks? The best thing one can wish for Carlo Stevo is that he die . . .

GIOVANNA: (*Standing up, seized with anger.*) And that would suit you just fine, I'm sure. And I almost pitied you! I told myself: this woman is like me, she is suffering . . . I hated you, but I pitied you, almost . . . A woman whom Carlo . . . This man, so difficult, so refined, a man for whom you're never dressed well enough or correctly enough . . . And I was timid . . . I got all dressed up for this visit . . . And what do I find but a sloppy woman, rude, some kind of factory worker wearing a shawl who is not ashamed to have been the cause of this mess . . .

MASSIMO: (*To Marcella.*) Leave her; she is suffering.

GIOVANNA: (*Insolently.*) Excuse me, I forgot that this is her house . . . (*To Massimo, with an awkward irony.*) I am sorry to be speaking that way about your friend in front of you, Signor.

MASSIMO: (*Casually.*) Don't worry about me, Signora Stevo.

MARCELLA: (*Standing up.*) You were protecting him against us, weren't you? You tried to wall him into his proper middle-class. You advised him to make his peace with the Ruler, to write nice books, something to pay for a little trip to Paris each year, or a new car. You took advantage of his sickness to kill in him the revolutionary, the hero, the apostle. Carlo always told me that marrying you was one of the worst consequences of his pneumonia.

GIOVANNA: He told you that? You?

MARCELLA: And who else would he say it to? Who else cares about Carlo Stevo's marriage? (*She sits down again and retreats into herself, head in her hands. In a doleful voice.*) I am crazy to bother with her tonight. Get her out of here, Massimo; tell her to go.

MASSIMO: (*To Giovanna, touching her arm.*) Enough of these women quarrels, Giovanna. Carlo often spoke of you to me during his stay in Vienna. He would say, "Vanna is beautiful, and she doesn't know that she is beautiful." He loved you more than you realize. He used to show your photograph and that of the child. He wanted to put the little girl in a sanatorium in Tyrol.

GIOVANNA: (*Softening, in spite of herself.*) And to think that he couldn't even make me a child who could walk like everybody else . . . If only he hadn't left me that cross to bear . . . I don't know you, Signor, but you saw a lot of my husband, you understand . . . One would think that she blames me for having nursed him. Of course, I nursed him. *I* didn't compromise him; *I* didn't get involved in politics. *I* didn't push him towards his downfall to get rid of him. And you must realize the situation that I'm in with a husband in prison, and my parents, whom I adore, but who are nevertheless, how shall I say? Because, well, I changed, while they, poor people . . . My father complaining that business is bad; my mother saying her rosary and playing the lottery every Saturday night. (*To Marcella, bitterly.*) Don't shrug your shoulders; you are a woman; you understand what I mean . . . The child, for example . . . Even before he went to prison, I was alone. Ah. Holy Virgin, do you think that is living? If at least I was the kind that could go and look for someone else! And when I come here tonight, I find you here with your lover . . .

MARCELLA: (*With a strained laugh.*) Ah, Massimo, this is absurd!

GIOVANNA: (*Insolently.*) Your boarder?

MARCELLA: (*Shaking her head.*) I don't rent that room anymore.

MASSIMO: (*Rising, tearing the headline from the newspaper lying on the table.*) Carlo Stevo has just retracted, in writing, what he calls his errors. He withdraws his accusations against certain heads of the party in power. His letter amounts to some sort of plea for mercy.

MARCELLA: (*Rising, shattered.*) It's not true!

MASSIMO: It's true, Marcella. It's already in all the evening papers.

MARCELLA: And you believe their lies? (*She grabs the newspaper.*)

MASSIMO: They showed me the letter.

MARCELLA: Who?

(*She keeps on reading avidly. He leans over her shoulder.*)

MASSIMO: It's true. For once, almost everything is true. The advice you gave your husband ended up by being followed, Signora Stevo.

(*Giovanna takes the newspaper that Marcella drops, and reads, leaning towards the lamp.*)

MARCELLA: (*Whispering.*) Massimo, how long have you known this?

MASSIMO: (*Whispering.*) Since this morning.

MARCELLA: (*Whispering.*) Why didn't you tell me anything?

MASSIMO: (*Whispering.*) Out of pity.

MARCELLA: (*Whispering, watching Giovanna.*) He really gave names? Which ones?

MASSIMO: (*Still whispering.*) Two or three compromised names. Don't worry; his letter embarrasses them more than it harms us. Don't make things worse,

Marcella. Give up your project; his position might well be atrocious, don't make things worse. Wait until we know what is what before you act.

MARCELLA: I didn't say anything.

MASSIMO: You are more transparent than you think.

GIOVANNA: (*Folding up the newspaper again, progressively happier.*) But then . . . So now, it means that . . . Thank God! . . . (*She puts on her gloves again, buttons up her coat, takes her purse and powders her face.*)

MASSIMO: (*Looking at her, to himself.*) Poor woman! She thinks she'll see him again soon.

GIOVANNA: Signora . . . Signor . . . (*To Massimo.*) Please don't bother; I'll find the door myself.

(*The doorbell rings.*)

MARCELLA: Already!

MASSIMO: That's not them; they wouldn't be ringing like that. But let me get it.

MARCELLA: I don't want them to find you here. Go into the other room.

(*The doorbell rings again. Giovanna sneers. Marcella closes the door behind Massimo who exits left, then goes towards the entry that opens on to the Via Fosca. She steps back seeing Alessandro.*)

GIOVANNA: (*With insolence.*) They don't rent rooms anymore.

MARCELLA: (*Emphasizing the word.*) My husband.

GIOVANNA: If he's got secrets to tell, I would advise him to speak low.

(*She exits, almost in a run. Alessandro takes off his raincoat and places it on a chair by the door. He walks into the lit zone of the room.*)

SCENE 2

ALESSANDRO: Who is that crazy woman?

MARCELLA: You know her. She's Carlo Stevo's wife.

ALESSANDRO: (*Observing her.*) I've arrived in the middle of a crisis. (*With a feeble attempt at humor.*) Perfect timing for a doctor. May I sit down?

MARCELLA: (*Standing.*) Yes.

ALESSANDRO: (*Sits down.*) You are beside yourself . . . What did that witch tell you?

MARCELLA: Nothing. She had come for news.

ALESSANDRO: And did you give her any?

MARCELLA: I only know what is in the evening papers. You've come to gloat, I suppose? You intend to observe the effect of this disaster on me? Well, it is not a disaster. You can leave reassured that I am not in pain.

ALESSANDRO: I have better reasons to see you.

MARCELLA: I don't want to know what they are.

ALESSANDRO: Well, I want you to know them. But first . . . (*He takes her hand.*) let me be sure that the Marcella I know is still alive.

MARCELLA: (*Violently withdrawing her hand.*) Enough, Alessandro. I want neither contacts nor consolations.

ALESSANDRO: Calm yourself. I do not intend to take you by surprise. (*After a slight pause.*) Did you ever wonder what became of me without you these last four years?

MARCELLA: I didn't have to wonder; you are on your way to becoming what you wanted to be—the eminent physician millionaires and celebrities obligatorily consult. You attended conferences; your photograph appeared prominently in *The Fascist Medical Journal, Year* X; you operated on an important member of the party, which allegedly earned you the invaluable favor of the big man himself. Is that it? I suppose that your bank account increased tenfold in four years. (*Sits down.*)

ALESSANDRO: (*He doesn't stop observing her and the room while speaking.*) I don't see why you can't congratulate me for living like a workman from the labor of his hands. (*He spreads his hands out complacently.*) The hands of a virtuoso, you used to call them when my skills as a surgeon used to interest you.

MARCELLA: And it's just that virtuosity that I hate. It did not take me long to understand that nothing counted for you except this ability you boast of. You don't care about science. Humanity . . .

ALESSANDRO: Spare me your big words.

MARCELLA: (*At first softly, then progressively more bitterly.*) I don't contest your talents, Alessandro, I have seen you at work myself. But your patients are only for you rich customers, fodder for success, an excuse for your experiments. Experimenting with the human body is your favorite pastime, even outside of surgery.

ALESSANDRO: Don't oversimplify everything, Marcella. With the human body, yes, and sometimes also with the human soul.

MARCELLA: (*In a slightly trembling voice.*) In any case, my own soul did not interest you.

ALESSANDRO: Are you sure? To tell the truth, the word is as outmoded in my vocabulary as in yours. Tell me more about myself, Marcella. I like seeing that you are still interested in my deeds and actions.

MARCELLA: (*Scathingly.*) What's left to say? You hunted at Grosseto with royalty. You smashed up against a wall, or traded or sold, two or three sports cars. You had two or three mistresses from among those flashy women wrapped in mink, whose names people whisper in restaurants and theaters as they walk by. You tired of them . . .

ALESSANDRO: That's a compliment to you.

MARCELLA: You sought from them, as you did from me, certain sensations, including that of danger. Come to think of it, we represent the same thing in your life as your Bugattis.

ALESSANDRO: (*Trying to turn the conversation into a joke.*) A way of getting there, what else?

MARCELLA: Yes, which explains why I soon got tired of being used as a vehicle. (*She sits down; in spite of everything, a sort of sensual intimacy is reigning between them.*)

ALESSANDRO: (*In the same tone.*) Speaking of speeding, I see you haven't forgotten the evening you chose to go on to San Marino on foot.

MARCELLA: I don't want to kill myself for nothing.

ALESSANDRO: (*Seriously.*) You reassure me. (*He rises and takes a few steps in the room.*) Do you know that I'd recognize you, with my eyes closed, by your way of speaking even if you disguised your voice? I can hear the influence of nineteenth-century poets, those profound imbeciles that cluttered up your father's mind and library, and whom you thought to find again in Carlo; my own influence, that at least taught you clarity, and . . . You haven't changed, Marcella.

MARCELLA: I can't say the same thing about you. You've aged.

ALESSANDRO: I've worn myself out. Believe me, old men don't wear themselves out; they preserve themselves. To wear out is the opposite of aging. Do you smoke?

MARCELLA: No.

ALESSANDRO: I see, cured of my vices. And what is this full ashtray doing here?

MARCELLA: (*Rising to take the ashtray and placing it on the chest of drawers.*) Don't waste your detective talents on such small stuff. I had lunch with a friend.

ALESSANDRO: The Iakovleff kid?

MARCELLA: You have me watched? What solicitude!

ALESSANDRO: I watch over you. It's more necessary than you think. Do you think that all you have to do to disappear is to bury yourself at the other end of Rome? It was not difficult to learn that a little seed vendor who needed to breathe fresher air abroad left you in charge of his business. Speaking of which, do you like this setting?

MARCELLA: It's not any different from the one I lived in before knowing you. To live a life without compromise is something.

ALESSANDRO: In that, my dear, I totally agree with you. (*He keeps on walking in the room, touching something here and there, picking up a book.*) What I have trouble understanding is how people like you, who lend the enemy a sort of superhuman malice, think that they are safe behind this ridiculous camouflage. Listen, how do you think you've been able to live here, more or less in peace, seemingly free, with the ideas and the friends you are known to have? At least give me credit for not having imposed myself on you these last four years.

MARCELLA: (*Bitterly.*) I see. I would be out on Lipari were it not for . . . I wonder what is behind this kindness. (*She sits down again.*)

ALESSANDRO: (*Also sitting down, softly.*) Nothing but the reluctance to see a woman end her days in a salt mine. My wife . . . Since our laws don't recognize divorce. And, without pretending that I think of you more often than I do, I admit that, from time to time, I wonder if I played my cards right . . .

MARCELLA: No question, you could have done better than to marry your nurse.

ALESSANDRO: My best nurse. No one has yet come close to you.

MARCELLA: Is that an offer of a job?

ALESSANDRO: (*Irritated.*) No, of course not. Neither is it an invitation to come back to the conjugal nest. Do you think I enjoyed that mixture of good times and trying ones, those outbursts of virtue of the romantic pulp heroine, those class rancors brought to bed . . .

MARCELLA: You liked it well enough to make me the Signora Sarte.

ALESSANDRO: (*Standing up.*) I know. I miscalculated, thinking marriage would make a woman settle down . . . When I think of all the family problems that decision brought me. Let it go. And even admitting that I was sometimes ineptly demanding or stupidly clever . . . You too connived. I realize that if I hadn't been in a position to do something for your father, that embittered failure you pass off as a great man, the ceremony would not have tempted you.

MARCELLA: (*Standing up, heatedly.*) You did nothing for him.

ALESSANDRO: After his dismissal, no. I had never committed myself to do so.

MARCELLA: (*In the same tone.*) And I guess it was to make me settle down that the day after the ceremony, as you call it, the minute we arrived in Cannes, you inflicted one of your former mistresses on me, that awful, overpainted Frenchwoman we met on the Croisette.

ALESSANDRO: (*In a soft ironic voice.*) Another compliment. There are few wives one is in such a hurry to introduce to a mistress.

MARCELLA: (*With much sadness.*) Please, Alessandro. Let's not reduce the past to pitiful bedroom squabbles. Politics drove us apart, that's all. Before that, I thought I loved you.

ALESSANDRO: No. Politics between a man and a woman is nothing more than a pretext. And furthermore, you know me. I wasn't foolish enough not to enroll in the party. And what's more, all hypocrisy notwithstanding, I rather admire this former mason who's trying to build up a nation. You accuse me of adulating success; on the other hand, you say that His success is fleeting . . . Granted. I'm only anticipating that time in history when this man, like all winners, will figure as a great loser. Meanwhile I don't deny bestowing my temporary esteem on practical results. Aren't you the least bit impressed by this man who made it?

MARCELLA: You forget that I saw how he made it. My father used to correct his first articles on the glories of socialism.

ALESSANDRO: Believe me, Marcella, doctrines one betrays are like women one abandons; they're always in the wrong. Was I going to compromise my hard-won position to fly to the aid of a handful of fanatics like your father or of visionaries like Carlo Stevo? One of the lessons experience taught me is that losers earn their defeat. But an objective view of political necessity is hardly what one can expect from the mistress of a martyr.

MARCELLA: I was not his mistress.

ALESSANDRO: I thought so. Don't you think I know Carlo? No one is better qualified than I to deliver his funeral oration tonight.

MARCELLA: What?

ALESSANDRO: (Nodding.) Yes. Carlo Stevo died on the island of Lipari about twenty-four hours ago.

MARCELLA: (Indignant.) And you didn't even have the courage to tell me the news straight out. They killed him?

ALESSANDRO: The word hardly applies to a sick man with no more than half a year to live. Say, rather, a kind of suicide. (Marcella doesn't say anything.) He got what he wanted. He . . . He was a dreamer, the word says it all for someone who knows that facts are not to be trifled with. Someone like Stevo could play only one role well, the role of a martyr. I hope that you notice that I don't even go on about his retraction; he could have been forced to make it, or it may be that a glimmer of good sense reached him before he died. We will never know; it doesn't matter. But in a way, the news moves me. We were friends before . . . Are you listening? (Marcella doesn't answer. In an irritated tone.) If you had asked my advice, I would have told you that you can't turn someone like Stevo into a man of action, any more than a swan can be turned into a bird of prey. You made a mistake, that's all. Since he met you, even on his many trips abroad when he got away from you for a time, friends said that he was not himself anymore. He was trying to be the hero you wanted him to be. When you're being watched by the regime, you don't launch some ridiculous coup d'état. And you don't divulge your plans to a Czech or Russian boyfriend met by chance in a Viennese restaurant—a friend, who, by the way, is a double agent.

MARCELLA: That's not true!

ALESSANDRO: Not that he did not suspect as much. Carlo wasn't stupid. But . . . He let you involve him in your plots, too happy, I imagine, to escape the need to think. Hounded by you, perhaps he willingly exposed himself to danger, out of weariness. As for the boy who hurried to join him back in Rome (I followed the whole thing quite closely), the boy you so generously welcomed, I would like to believe that gathering information at your expense was not his sole aim . . . One couldn't be around Carlo without loving him. One can't be around you without loving you. And if the boy didn't warn you that the trap was closing in, perhaps it was because there was no more time. And how could he admit to those he loved that he had at first betrayed them? And your dear Massimo needs the police money to support a mistress.

MARCELLA: It's a lie! It's a lie!

ALESSANDRO: I assure you. One of my patients. A little woman with a rather faded look. Does that shock you? It would be funny if you were in love with him.

MARCELLA: (*Controlling herself, in a derisive tone.*) Is that all? Let's get back to Carlo Stevo's death. If you have more details don't hide them from me.

ALESSANDRO: I would advise you not to let your imagination run away with you. I am telling you what I was told. (*In a softer tone.*) I had a telephone call not long ago, while I was getting ready to go to the reception at the Palazzo Balbo. The news will be kept secret for a few days. Still, I thought it would be better if I . . .

MARCELLA: (*Fighting tears.*) Thank you. (*She starts sobbing.*)

ALESSANDRO: Well, my dear, and I thought you would not forgive him his retraction.

MARCELLA: (*In exalted tones.*) They wrung that letter out of him. A moment of weakness, the lapse of a dying man . . . But don't you see that everything has been erased, explained, paid for. Just go and be a big success tonight by insulting our martyrs!

ALESSANDRO: (*Exasperated, laying his cards on the table.*) Enough! Enough of these big words, Marcella! Don't be obstinate. Don't make this wretched man into a hero. You admitted yourself that you were never lovers. Now you're alone again. Alone, night and day . . Let me tell you that there isn't a single minute of our married life that I don't miss, even the quarrels, even the scenes. You are not going to remain buried here among these grubs? Do you remember our first date, a fall Sunday in Reggiomonte? You loved me that day . . .

MARCELLA: I was crazy about you.

ALESSANDRO: It's the same thing.

(*He grabs her face between his hands and tries to kiss her. She draws away and moves back towards the back of the room.*)

MARCELLA: (*In a shattered voice.*) Stay where you are.

ALESSANDRO: You are afraid? You are afraid of yourself?

MARCELLA: I'm still in love with you. And you know it. But it's all over between us.

(*A pause. Marcella takes a comb and combs her hair.*)

ALESSANDRO: (*Going near the bed standing at the edge of the shadows. In a soft voice.*) Is this where you sleep?

MARCELLA: (*In a toneless voice.*) Yes.

ALESSANDRO: (*Caresses the blanket with his fingertips moving up to the pillow. Suddenly in alarm.*) Well! I see you sleep better with this gun under your pillow? (*He takes the weapon and examines it with curiosity.*) I recognize it. Well kept. Is it loaded?

MARCELLA: (*Grabbing it away from him.*) In any case not for you. Your death would benefit no one.

ALESSANDRO: (*Looking at her carefully.*) I seem to remember that once, when you were no doubt convinced that humanity had to be served till the end, you used to condemn suicide . . .

MARCELLA: (*Interrupting him.*) I don't condemn it anymore. Too many people are driven to it. But there are other ways of dying.

ALESSANDRO: Such as? (*Marcella doesn't say anything. He starts again, in a low voice.*) Am I right in remembering that your father saw political assassinations as the only recourse of oppressed people? (*In a slightly demented gesture Marcella puts a finger to her lips. Her pale face must look like the face of the Medusa. After a pause, sarcastically.*) And so this scheme is not even of your own making? That's women for you!

MARCELLA: If I act, it will be more than a scheme.

ALESSANDRO: What you have in mind is more difficult than you imagine. The security police aren't there for nothing. He exposes himself less than the press would like to make us believe.

MARCELLA: He is speaking tonight at Palazzo Balbo.

ALESSANDRO: (*Shaken, in spite of himself.*) You cannot fool me. You are trying to trip me up. When one is thinking about doing it, one doesn't advertise.

MARCELLA: I trust you in a certain way.

ALESSANDRO: Marcella, your project is stupid.

(*He makes a gesture to take again the gun which she slips into the drawer of the table, locking it. Then she remains standing, hands on the oilcloth tablecloth.*)

MARCELLA: (*With disdain.*) I know you'll do nothing to interfere with my plans. Admit it: destruction fascinates you. You're too curious about the human soul, as you say, not to want to know if I'll go all the way or not. And, what's more, you would feel like a fool calling the police to say that your wife is going to kill Julius Caesar in an hour.

ALESSANDRO: Caesar did not make me responsible for his welfare. Do you know how to shoot?

MARCELLA: (*Amused.*) Don't you remember?

ALESSANDRO: (*Also now amused.*) Of course. (*Seriously, in a persuasive tone.*) Listen, Marcella. A guard will grab your arm; the shot will miss or hit some bystander in the crowd. Tomorrow the newspapers will praise His courage in the face of danger. Some poor devils will be arrested, paying for your grand gesture. A few foreigners will be kicked out. Is that your goal? Are you so set on being shot, point blank, by a guard, or knocked senseless, or beaten to death in a police station?

MARCELLA: What a nuisance for you. After all, I officially bear your name.

ALESSANDRO: (*To himself.*) She's crazy. She's crazy, and right now, she hates me. I mustn't push her too far. And indeed, my name . . . (*To Marcella.*) Do you think Carlo Stevo would have approved?

MARCELLA: (*Thinking it over for a moment.*) I don't know. It doesn't matter.

ALESSANDRO: (*To himself.*) I must win time. Tension like this can't last. I should stay with her. Hold her back against her will . . . No. (*To Marcella.*) How long have you been planning this?

MARCELLA: Forever, it seems to me.

ALESSANDRO: And this is why you took that gun from me when you left Reggiomonte?

MARCELLA: (*Sitting down again at the table.*) I don't know anymore . . . Ideas come and go, then come back, then they stay on . . . But what bothers me is . . . this old theft . . . (*In a half joking tone.*) Here, let's settle up. Render unto Caesar . . . (*She opens an old wallet lying on the table, and takes out two or three bills haphazardly, some coins which she pushes towards him.*)

ALESSANDRO: (*To himself.*) Let's play along. (*To Marcella, picking up a coin.*) If you insist, Marcella. I accept this because when someone gives you a knife he asks for a coin; otherwise, the gift brings bad luck, the same holds true for a gun. Is that all you have left?

MARCELLA: It's more than I need.

ALESSANDRO: (*Getting ready to leave, putting on his raincoat.*) Promise me something, Marcella. I won't try to dissuade you; the whole business would start again tomorrow, if I did, or the day after tomorrow, or in a week. Take that walk; go to the Palazzo Balbo—if you can get through the mob, test your resolution and strength. I have my own ideas about freedom. But if opportunity, courage, or faith fail you, (believe me, there is no faith worth killing for, even less dying for), remember that someone will be there, in those pompous, ugly rooms, on the other side of the lit-up balcony, among the throng and the footmen proffering drinks; someone only too happy to applaud the action *you will not carry out.* After the speech, if nothing happens, I'll stand near the Corso, on the left side of the street, in front of the Theater Mondo.

MARCELLA: (*With a strained laugh.*) Ready to escort me back?

ALESSANDRO: (*In a serious tone.*) Yes, for life. (*He puts his hand on the handle of the left door which he opens slightly.*)

MARCELLA: Not that way.

ALESSANDRO: (*After stealing a glance towards the door she shuts again.*) Excuse me. (*She walks before him towards the entry. They stop, squeezed one against the other on what is supposed to be the threshold of the door opening on the Via Fosca. They are facing a dark spot. He goes on in a low voice.*) Remember that you used to condemn suicide. This is suicide. You don't stand a chance.

MARCELLA: My life is not worth more than that.

ALESSANDRO: I've been offered a job in England. Maybe we could . . .

MARCELLA: (*In an almost tender tone.*) No. All I'm asking you is not to betray me.

ALESSANDRO: (*Speaking more loudly.*) Do you take me for your Russian student? (*He leaves. Turning around to face her.*) Tonight, ten thirty. Across from the Theater Mondo. (*She walks towards the center of the room again. He takes a few steps to the right, along the footlights. To himself.*) Crazy? No. A heroine? Fool, I'm almost hoping it happens . . . Could it be, tonight, during the speech, on Piazza Balbo. Nonsense. Melodrama! (*He disappears.*)

SCENE 3

MARCELLA: I'll never see him again. (*She takes a few steps in the room.*) How slowly time passes! One more hour, rather two, especially if . . . (*She dunks a washcloth in the water pitcher and presses it against her face.*) My hands aren't shaking. That's a good sign. I should change clothes . . . This broken strap . . . (*She goes near the door on the left, hesitates.*) I wonder if Alessandro thought, a little while back, that . . . Could that boy still be there? Impossible. (*She knocks lightly on the door.*) Are you there?

MASSIMO'S VOICE: (*In a whisper.*) Yes.

MARCELLA: (*Uncertain.*) Wait. I'll join you. (*She hesitates, her hand on the door handle. To herself.*) Eavesdropping? It's disgusting; he's one of them. Alessandro's information is never wrong. Or rather no; he *was* one of them. And so what? I should be outraged. No. Freed from conventions . . . (*Opening the door.*) After all, I am entitled to spend my last hour with whomever I please. (*She walks into the room on the left.*)

(*A white and cold light coming from the street lamps outside, creeps in through an unseen window.*)

SCENE 4

There is only one bed in this room; its headboard faces the audience. Massimo is lying on it, on a bare mattress. Next to the bed, a straw chair. A low table on which there is a pile of folded blankets. These few props are meant to suggest an unfurnished room after someone has moved out.

MASSIMO: (*Raising himself, leaning on an elbow.*) I heard everything.

MARCELLA: (*Standing on the right. In a sad voice.*) You were spying on us?

MASSIMO: Yes . . . No . . . Let's say I didn't want to leave without seeing you again. (*Marcella moans softly.*) Don't cry. Look, I'm not crying. And don't blush either. After all, it's dark, anyway. (*In an almost low voice.*) You love him. You love THIS MAN FROM ANOTHER WORLD? In spite of yourself. You gave away your secret for nothing to this insolent fool who is so sure of not being crazy like the rest of us, so sure of seeing the world as it really is . . . Oh, don't worry; he doesn't believe it. He was afraid for a moment, but he doesn't believe it.

MARCELLA: Since I told him about it, I believe it a little less myself.

MASSIMO: But I believed it, really, I have believed it since I understood certain awkward questions about the firing range of weapons, and certain silences, and that air of being sure that you will be able to pull it off, all by yourself. You didn't tell me anything that I didn't already know. And you yourself had guessed this black spot in my past, hadn't you? My past, what a silly expression when one isn't even twenty-two yet. You don't pick up a stray dog without realizing that he is full of vermin.

MARCELLA: Am I accusing you? Everything would have turned out the same without you. (*She sits down on the chair near the bed. For a while neither speaks. Then.*)

MASSIMO: (*Thoughtfully.*) It's hard, isn't it, the death of someone?

MARCELLA: What's even harder is that he gave in before dying. But the point I'm at, it doesn't matter.

MASSIMO: Hatred . . . Your hatred . . . When a man and a woman insult each other the way you did a little while back, it's obvious they love each other. And did you hear her, that woman filled with hatred who loved Carlo? Your hatred . . . Oh, I know, it's not that you lack reasons: your father—it's strange that one can't talk of avenging a father without seeming to be part of an old melodrama—and Carlo, and the other one, the hero of you all, the poor man who was bumped off on the banks of the Tiber—you know who I mean—he is also unavenged. And even if there were no other reasons than to put an end to these lies scribbled in large letters on the walls, to stifle that voice doling out swill to the crowds . . . But that's not it . . . You want to kill Caesar, but even more, you want to kill Alessandro, and me, and yourself. Wipe the slate clean . . . Leave the nightmare behind. Shoot, as in a theater, to bring down the set behind the smoke. Do away with these people who do not exist.

MARCELLA: (*In a tired voice.*) It's simpler than that. When I was a nurse in Bologna I was always the one who did the dirty work no one else would do. Somebody has to do what others don't have the courage to.

MASSIMO: (*Continuing.*) . . . and who do not exist. Does he exist, that hollow drum beaten by the fears of a class and the vanities of a people? Do you exist? Are you going to kill to try to feel real? And Carlo who fought them, gave in, then begged for mercy, then perhaps did what he had to do to escape the need for mercy—was he real? We are all shreds of torn cloths, faded rags, bits of compromises. The cherished disciple is not the one asleep on the Master's shoulder in the paintings, but the one who hanged himself with thirty pieces of silver in his pocket. Or rather no; they are one man, one and the same man. Like people who in dreams think they are someone else. You dream of killing or of being killed; you shoot, and it is yourself you are shooting at. The shot wakes you up; that's what death is like. Waking us up is death's way of reaching us . . . Will you wake up in an hour? Will you understand that killing is impossible, that dying is impossible?

MARCELLA: (Stifling a yawn.) But how? If I miss him, they won't miss me.

MASSIMO: (Getting excited.) And you take your knife, Charlotte, and you climb into the coach for Paris, and you strike deep, like a butcher, right to the heart. Ah, killing, giving birth, you're all good at that, you women, at all those bloody operations. And your sacrifice saves no one, on the contrary. Formerly, Christian women used to go to the temples to spit on idols to make sure of being killed. And public law and order were preserved, as you well know; the women were wiped out, and then chapels that looked like temples were built on their tombs. This man, this false god, you won't kill him. And if he dies, he triumphs; his death is Caesar's apotheosis. But you don't care. This is the only way you can scream "No" when everyone is saying "Yes." Ah, I love you. I who would never have enough courage, or faith, or hope to do what you are doing, I love you. My saint, my Fury, hatred that is our love, vengeance that is all we have of justice, let me kiss the hands that will not shake . . .

(He leans over, takes her hands, kisses them. She withdraws them quickly but in a gesture that grazes his face softly like a caress.)

MARCELLA: Don't go off on a tangent to make me forget what I have in mind. The letter?

MASSIMO: What about it?

MARCELLA: They showed it to you. Therefore you're still in contact with them.

MASSIMO: Carlo knew it. Do you think one can escape that tangle so quickly? I protected the both of you more than you think.

MARCELLA: (With a bitter laugh.) You, too!

MASSIMO: What are you doing?

MARCELLA: (Lifting her arm, trying to tell the time by her watch in the weak light coming from outside.) I'm looking at the time. I don't want to go too early, to have to wait in the piazza and be noticed. I still have time. (Leaning back she puts her head on the pillow, half lying on the bed. Little by little, she will stretch out completely.)

MASSIMO: Would you like to sleep? Do you want me to wake you up?

MARCELLA: No. I don't trust you that much. (*After a pause.*) Did you know about Carlo's death?

MASSIMO: (*In a soft voice.*) I learned it only a few hours ago . . . But I was expecting it more than you.

MARCELLA: Do you think they killed him?

MASSIMO: Who knows? Enough . . . Leave it alone . . .

MARCELLA: You see that I'm right to go tonight.

MASSIMO: (*Thoughtfully.*) No. All in all, no. I want you to live.

MARCELLA: (*In an almost lighthearted tone, deliberately speaking of something else.*) Do you know what I'm thinking of? Of your complicated inventions. Of the false picture you painted with a little bit of truth . . . Alessandro . . . And you . . . And even Carlo. My father's death, for example. I am not really this heroic daughter that Alessandro imagines. And Sandro . . . Yes, I loved him, I missed him, and I fought missing him. But maybe sensual love is not as important as one thinks . . .

MASSIMO: (*Eagerly.*) Isn't that so?

MARCELLA: (*To herself.*) I'm lying. Even so close to death I'm lying. And nothing is simple at the same time, even though I love Sandro, I . . . To think that sometimes I couldn't even bring myself to look at him . . . What's he doing with that sick girl? If only I could be caressed by his hands, pull myself up a little on the pillow so that his head would touch my breast . . . Too bad, that will never happen.

MASSIMO: (*Slowly, with bitterness.*) For nothing . . . You are going there for nothing. They'll lie about everything; they will turn it all to their advantage, even you attempted revenge. Tomorrow they'll say: a madwoman, a demented person, the wife of a certain eminent doctor S. who . . . A little more mud thrown on Carlo. And me, they'll also use me to blacken you.

MARCELLA: (*Withdrawing her hand.*) Is that my fault?

(*After a pause.*)

MASSIMO: I would really like you to understand. Imagine a child who learned about hunger, war, escape, being arrested at the border . . . a boy who had seen everything, but didn't suffer . . . For a child, it's a game. A student who misses classes, who takes the money that he's offered here and there . . . Who keeps on playing with life and death . . . A boy inured to everything . . . "Like those who have no hope." The day I met you I understood. Perhaps you will change the world since you changed me.

MARCELLA: (*Tenderly.*) No, I didn't change you. You are what you are. (*While he spoke, he slowly got up. Now she also rises, puts her hand on his shoulder.*) Listen, a little while ago with Alessandro, I forgot Carlo and what I am going to do tonight. And why? Back to the old game of quarrels and love scenes. Oh, only for one second, but more than once, several times . . . I am neither cleaner nor purer than you.

MASSIMO: (*Passionately, in a low voice.*) Do you know, sometimes I think that we're the ones who are not pure, we who have been humiliated, stripped, sullied, who without ever having had anything, have lost everything, we who have no country, no party (no, no, don't deny it!) we could be the ones through whom the Kingdom will come. We are the ones they can't corrupt anymore, the ones they can't deceive. Let's start right now . . . by ourselves. A world so different that it will make all the others fall, a world without street riots, without violence, without lies, especially without lies. But it will be a world where people would not kill.

MARCELLA: (*Not listening, softly.*) You are like a child. And that is why I trust you, because you seem like a child. (*She stretches, like a woman waking up. In a confidential tone.*) When I was living with Alessandro, I wanted a child. A child by Sandro . . . Can you imagine: raised in a den for young Fascists. No, thank God . . . There are better ways of giving birth to the future.

MASSIMO: (*Changing moods, exasperated.*) The future . . . Ah, you've aggravated me enough, you and Carlo with your future generation, your future society, your future, your beautiful future. Your poor refuge for the persecuted . . . Look at the people in the street later, when you go out there, and ask yourself if they're the ones you build your future on. There is no future. There is only a man you want to kill, who, dead, will rise again like a target in a shooting gallery, a man who thinks he can shape the future by banging his fists. And you noticed, the other day, his two important guests, General Goering and Colonel Von Papen, they also have their little ideas about the future. And Carlo, dead, disgraced, having perhaps stopped believing in the future, and you with your pitiful fifteen minutes of future . . . Or, rather, no. (*He also leans over his wrist to tell the time. In a different, practical tone.*) Twenty to ten. You'll never be able to get through to the front row. It seems to me that you should put it off till tomorrow, your act that will save the future.

MARCELLA: (*Getting up.*) You think you're so clever. Do you think I would tell Alessandro the exact time, the exact place. I'm going to wait by the exit on the little Piazza San Giovanni-Martire. There's a corner with a statue.

MASSIMO: (*Tenderly.*) So you, too, were playing two games at once. (*Unnoticeably, she moves away.*) In that case, lie down again. You still have a whole hour left.

MARCELLA: (*Going towards the door on the right.*) Give up. You did your best to make everything go wrong. You know that a person has only a limited amount of strength and that I've almost used up mine. But don't you see that my whole life, even our moment of intimacy tonight, is grotesque if I don't do it? One would think that you envy my courage.

MASSIMO: (*Getting up.*) You don't have the courage not to do it. Would you like me to go in your place?

MARCELLA: (*With affectionate disdain.*) You! (*He feels along the wall, turns on the switch for a lightbulb hanging from the ceiling. She takes a step towards him.)* There is something I would like to know before I go. Carlo never said anything about you . . . It's . . . It's like a sort of betrayal on his part.

MASSIMO: *(In a light tone.)* Ah! These jealousies between disciples . . . How could I know? Leave those old stories alone. *(He lights a cigarette. After a pause.)* My turn to ask a question. A little while back, that crazy woman . . . It wasn't because of your husband that she sneered.

MARCELLA: You know better than anyone else that she was lying.

MASSIMO: Is that a reproach?

MARCELLA: If you were trying to send me there, you could not have found a better way to do it.

(She goes into the next room dimly lit by the night lamp. She can be half seen leaning over a table, opening a drawer, wrapping a shawl around herself. Massimo turns out the lights in the left room and joins her. In the almost total darkness, they can be barely seen going towards the door opening on to the Via Fosca.)

MASSIMO: *(Suddenly.)* Carlo would not have approved of a crime.

MARCELLA: *(Trying to understand.)* What crime? *(Then heatedly.)* Shut up! What do you know about it?

MASSIMO: *(Bitterly, to himself.)* That's true. She knew him better than I did.

SCENE 5

The two characters reappear center stage, near the footlights, walking along what stands for a street in Rome. A radio in a building somewhere blares out a popular love song. Marcella turns towards Massimo.

MARCELLA: *(Bitingly.)* When I came in, back there . . . weren't you afraid . . . that I would shoot you first?

MASSIMO: Not too much. The point you're at, one doesn't deviate.

(They take a few steps together. She stops.)

MARCELLA: Tell me goodbye. *(She kisses him. They hug. Then, as though waking up from a dream.)* We mustn't be seen together. Where are you going?

MASSIMO: *(Hesitating.)* Nowhere . . . As usual . . .

(He disappears in the darkness. Marcella takes a few steps towards the right, going towards the back of the stage. Now the radio is blaring out the speech of the Dictator. His voice will be heard throughout the scene, more and more loudly and more and more indistinctly. Only a few words can be made out, continuously repeated, drowned out by cheers.)

VOICE OF THE DICTATOR: To impose on the world . . . The future of a great nation . . . Subversive ideologies . . . Out of date liberalism . . . Power . . . Out of date ideologies . . . To impose on the world . . . When the refuge of liberal ideas will be swept into the gutters . . . A subversive liberalism . . . Soldier virtues . . . Our glorious ancestors . . . Our Conquests . . . Old fashioned ideologies . . . The future of the Empire . . . Through strength . . . The Empire of the future . . .

MARCELLA: (*Walking faster and faster.*) Make that voice shut up. Make that voice . . . Go, run . . . (*The sound of rain patter is heard. The sound of the storm mingles with that of the radio in a growing, deafening noise.*) The storm . . . The storms protect you . . . Enough! Enough! Enough! Shoot that voice. Faster . . . Careful not to slip.

(*She exits running. The deafening noise continues. A shot is heard, followed by a series of shots. The radio, still almost intelligible, goes on.*)

VOICE OF THE RADIO: You have just heard . . . Here R.V.E. Radio Eternal City. The speech of the Dictator. Palazzo Balbo. Tomorrow's program . . . Reception at Palazzo Balbo . . . Tomorrow . . .

(*Total darkness.*)

ACT III

SCENE 1

In front of the Theater Mondo. The set is made up of two enormous posters harshly lit, placed in the foreground, showing pictures of Angiola Fides. Between the two posters, slightly further back, the box office of an invisible cashier.

ALESSANDRO: *(Alone, leaning against the poster on the left.)* Up to now, I never knew what the word "waiting" meant. Waiting for what? You fool! All you did was walk through the gilded reception rooms filled with uniforms and evening clothes; you went out again, you worked your way up to the front rows of the crowd; you waited. With irony, with anxiety, with an inept enthusiasm you didn't think yourself capable of. . . What were you waiting for? You don't hate Him; you don't want His death; after all, you understand those politicians who try to keep people in line; the most you strive for is to be neither fooled nor victimized. And yet, admit it, from one of His clichés to the next, from raised fist to raised fist, you feared, hoped, despaired, that a shot would ring out. But nothing happened . . . The imperial dummy withdrew from the balcony, safe and sound, not even dampened by the rain. The crowd disbanded in the storm. Did you really think that *something* would emerge out of this inertia, this apathy, these orchestrated ovations, *that Someone* . . . And that *Someone* would be her . . . And like a pagan defending a Christian woman thrown to the beasts in the circus, you were ready for one of these great moments that occur in films or books. For you really don't love her that much . . . That's not what you want; you have enough good sense not to wish for more chaos in this already chaotic world.

Well then, what? The feeling that this play can't go on, that this precarious, ramshackle house will crumble one day, and that it would be a fine thing that She be the one, that She be the woman who . . . Here you are, reduced to the role of an operatic character, of a silly lover, of a romantic conspirator. And you stand under this movie awning like a man looking for a one-night mistress, but She doesn't show up either at this appointment after defeat you had given her, Via Fosca. You better watch . . .

(A few people, walking by the posters one after the other, buy tickets. Angiola Fides is the last one to arrive; she is wearing a dark coat over a thin pink dress.)

ANGIOLA FIDES: (At the box office.) One loge, please.

(She also disappears between the posters. The usher guides her with a little red flashlight aimed towards the ground.)

THE USHER: Careful, Madam, there's a step.
ALESSANDRO: (Turning his head away.) No. No one . . . Gawkers, the same ones who a while back were cheering the man on the balcony. This time attracted by a talking picture . . . Or wanting to get out of the rain, like I'm pretending to do. But her? But that face I held between my hands just a little while ago, that face offered to something else besides love, and which was also faking? You pictured your wife, your mistress, the nurse you used to take for rides in your little Fiat on Sundays, in the outskirts of Bologna, as a heroine, a Charlotte Corday? But what if they suspected her, arrested her just as She was . . . No, you would know about it already, news like that travels quickly in the crowd. And what if she came on Piazza Balbo, and if courage gave out at the last minute? She would be here, looking for me; she would be reduced once again, to a woman looking for comfort. But no, she staged the classical scene for you: vanity, hysterics, lies. Ridiculed. And that noise in the next room . . . That was the other one, the little comrade who was perhaps listening, the cheap prop of her melodrama. You are compromised . . . No! They are too compromised themselves to compromise you . . . And how are you going to manage now, without a car, and not even a taxi in sight? Will you walk home in the rain? Face your furniture, your rugs, the last issue of the *International Surgery Review*? Of course not; you will wait, nailed to the spot. You want to wait. I'll give you ten more minutes.

(The stage goes dark then light comes on immediately again. The set consists of one single loge box in the middle of the stage. Angiola Fides is sitting there, seen from her profile, her hand on the red velvet border of the loge, her black coat thrown on the back of her seat. She is looking towards the left at a screen that we don't see, in a part of the room that we also don't see.)

ANGIOLA: (*To herself.*) It was pointless, this ride through Rome to look for what? But since Sir Junius preferred not to go out tonight . . . He is tired. This morning, he visited the Vatican Museum . . . A foreigner's notion . . . And furthermore, he steers clear of political events; one never knows how these things turn out. But I hungered for the streets of Rome . . . And yet, when one has seen Paris or New York . . . And I wasn't keen on showing Sir Junius Stein's chauffeur that I know by heart all these poor neighborhoods . . . I had forgotten that Via Fosca was that short. And when I entered the courtyard of number eleven (the same garbage can on the left, still in the same spot, as though it hadn't been emptied in six years) this fat, unkempt woman: "What are you doing here? This isn't a house for the likes of you, my little lady . . ." Too well dressed. I should have, at least, left my rings in the hotel. (*She touches them with affection.*) And even if I had gone up the stairs, if I had knocked, then what? First of all, perhaps they no longer live there . . . But let's suppose that the old man had opened the door or Rosalie . . . I couldn't very well take them to the Caesar Palace, be photographed with them by the reporters . . . The Movie Star Angiola Fides between her old father and her sister . . . Touching . . . No, they never helped me to leave that slum, on the contrary. I got out all alone; I help no one. Sir Junius is not a philanthropic institution. (*Total darkness. The stage is now only lit by the ray of light coming from the projectionist. Angiola's words are half drowned out by the soundtrack of the film being shown.*) But what you wanted was to come here all alone, in this loge. Incognito. You sense all these people in the darkness, these people who have come here to watch you; they are settling in their seats . . . Not counting those who came for the earlier showing and who stayed to watch you again. And among these men, there are perhaps some who, on summer nights when you'd escape Rosalia's watchful eyes, would take you for a slut in the street, for a poor man's whore. Well, you are taking your revenge on Via Fosca. You went through some hard times, starving with your actor, until the day the director of the R.A.F. took a liking to you . . . Even now, life is not all fun . . . But there is this woman now seen on all the screens in the world, this woman they desire, and of whom they dream and who makes them weary of their own wives. You are going to see her. You have an appointment with yourself here. You are going to see yourself, Angiola . . . (*Sounds and noises from a documentary about current events.*) No, it's not you yet. Some news or other. Japanese troops in Mongolia . . . Soldiers, tanks . . . Like in old war movies. Jews beaten in Germany . . . Too bad . . . Spring fashions from Paris . . .

VOICE OF THE USHER: Careful, Sir, there's a step.

ALESSANDRO: (*Settling in a seat.*) Excuse me.

(*He sits down next to Angiola. The red light from the usher's flashlight goes out.*)

ALESSANDRO: (*To himself.*) I must think clearly . . . I must reflect, go into myself . . . Alone in the dark, in the emptiness . . . No need to look at the screen . . . No, not quite alone: a woman. But, she is not bothering you, after all. What? That voice screaming . . . Look . . . The movie of your life being shown backwards; flags flowing, a balcony . . . Are you going to expect again a gun shot to punctuate each sentence? Of course not; one doesn't shoot ghosts . . Besides, it's old news, last week's. A surgeons' convention: I am there myself among those men all looking alike, those black and white dots. General Goering is in Rome . . .

ANGIOLA: (*To herself.*) . . . is in Rome. The Chief of State on the train platform . . . People are right to say that the Chief of State is very courteous. When I was presented to him; when he praised in me a new star . . . We are ruled by a genius . . . This man next to me is very attractive . . . He must be coming from a party. A man of the world. The train arriving brings Colonel Von Papen . . .

ALESSANDRO: (*To himself.*) Enough! Enough of this rehash of news items, of these bits of film created by *God and Universe Incorporated.* Look elsewhere . . . This red light: EMERGENCY EXIT. There is no exit. What does that red light remind you of? The lamp before the Madonna that she keeps out of habit, or because it looks good to her neighbors. Or maybe Iakovleff has a liking for icons. And they sit or lie down under that lamp, and they are making fun of me, that fool . . . Cartoons: clowns rushing around like the thoughts in my mind during that wretched wait. How strange: I never understood before these crude mechanisms, these tricks of sound. But here, at least one knows one is being fooled, one doesn't expect anything. That clown falls, stumbling like me, a while back, against an absent woman . . . And now something else: tragedy: an enormous woman's head slowly revolving like the globe, and the bone structure like imperceptible hollows, everything that one sees when close to a loved face . . . Remember her just a short time ago . . . Beautiful without make-up, beautiful in spite of her worn hands, her working woman dress . . . An equal, an adversary, something to turn you off forever from the pretty whores of the Signora Speranza. Stop it . . . Forget about her. The woman on the screen is lovely too, thanks, of course, to make-up and lighting. She is dancing . . . A shoulder, a half bared breast showing on the empty rectangle. You have always thought that flesh was the only reality, the only recourse. Even shadow flesh . . .

(*The stage gets darker and darker.*)

ANGIOLA: (*To herself.*) That man is looking at me. Or rather, he is looking at Angiola Fides . . . Algenib, since in this film, that is my name . . . In a palace, with her father, this venerable sheik wearing a burnoose . . . Not your own father, not at all venerable, the ruined count living at the expense of rich relatives . . . And this kind black woman kneeling to put on your shoes, and she protects you when a big snake . . . Not your boring Rosalia in her gray cloth dress . . . Algenib under palm trees by the sea . . . But your own youthful days of venturing, half-dressed, on the beach came quickly to an end. You were placed in a convent by a cousin who was more than willing to pay for your education, but not so willing for her son to . . . And your first lover, Algenib, Lord Southsea . . . How handsome he was, at least on the screen, for in the flesh, Jim Taylor . . . And you are dancing, and Lord Southsea kills a man who insulted you in a bar . . . All men love you, even those who insult you . . . Now the agent of the foreign power tracks you, like a handsome prey . . . But all you had, yourself, was Paolo Farina who married you, the fool, after Tonio de Trapani dropped you like a coward . . . And then, of course, all the others, your rotten actor, and sir Junius who is trying to have your marriage annulled in Rome . . . but no one strolled in fields of flowers with you, no one sailed in a bark . . . And your secret agent forces you to break in, at night, during a ball, into the office of the Residence, to steal state documents . . . And you are searching, leaning over a desk in your long white crepe sheath, and your hair flows on your chest like a silk fringe . . . And your chest is heaving because you are afraid. You had to take that pose many times before the director was satisfied. And you start, feeling Lord Southsea's hand on your shoulder . . .

(*Total darkness.*)

ALESSANDRO: (*To himself.*) This young woman next to me looking avidly at this inept scene. Beautiful . . . This naked arm, so close . . . A reality . . . Put your fingers on this shoulder, touch it, as if by chance, as if in a dream . . . so that she can't tell for sure . . . She is not drawing away, imperceptibly leaning towards me . . . Press your hand a little harder . . . Caress her, this woman alive among those ghosts . . . Like on the screen, the gesture of the actor . . . Feel the thin material . . . Ah, to forget this tumult, this madness in another madness, another tumult . . . Please, signora, a little moment of forgetfulness . . . And she is willing, and you know that she is willing, that she is giving in . . . Easy . . . Experienced . . . What pleasure to do without the words, even without the kiss that the actor there . . . This close-up of a kiss which is nothing but a symbol of the rest . . . She knows her stuff . . .

ANGIOLA: (*To herself.*) Don't hold out . . . You like it . . . In the dark, in the back of this loge . . . No one will know . . . Nothing to fear . . . He finds you beautiful . . . He wants Algenib . . . But you are Algenib . . . Give in . . . Be soft . . .

ALESSANDRO: (*To himself.*) The screen like a mirror reflecting a couple . . . Underneath the thin silk, the sweet, the hard flesh . . . Delicious examination of a body . . . Not so different from the one a doctor . . . And this shudder, this spasm, this letting-go, not so different from those of a patient. Push this idea away; it spoils your pleasure . . . Concentrate on this warmth, on this hand moving on you like an underwater plant . . . How many in this room, at this moment? Flower, spring, garden . . . Ah, the only thing that is clean, totally certain, the only satisfaction, the only . . .

ANGIOLA: (*To herself.*) The lovers are fleeing pursued by the British police . . . The boat tips, the wave falls back . . . The sea is spent . . . Lacy foam . . The lovers sink together . . .

ALESSANDRO: (*To himself.*) . . . Sink together . . . A while back, you wanted to die for . . . The movie ends on an ecstatic organ chord . . . And in one minute, the lights . . . It doesn't matter; I owe this woman the only good moment of the day.

(*After a while, the lights go on. Alessandro and Angiola can be seen, standing next to each other, getting ready to leave.*)

ALESSANDRO: (*With courtesy.*) Signora . . .

ANGIOLA: (*Very polite.*) Signor . . . (*To herself.*) I was right; he is handsome. And it's the best thing I had since arriving in Rome. See him again? One never knows what one is getting into. Better not spoil a good memory.

ALESSANDRO: (*To himself.*) Elegant . . . A foreigner for sure . . . Like so many others, she does her best to look like Angiola Fides. A prostitute? No, a woman who likes to love . . . Shall I take this further? One never knows what one is getting into. Better not spoil a good memory. (*After hesitating a little, to Angiola.*) American?

ANGIOLA: (*Faking a British accent.*) No, English . . . Are you Italian?

ALESSANDRO: (*Moved, searching for his words, in a low voice, in English.*) Thank you, love. It was wonderful.

ANGIOLA: (*Putting on lipstick, keeping the British accent.*) Wasn't it? Don't think, my dear, that I'm like that with everybody.

ALESSANDRO: (*Irritated.*) I don't expect excuses.

(*They take a few steps towards the exit. The light goes out then immediately goes on again showing them outside, between the two posters. A few other spectators also come out.*)

ANGIOLA: (*Continuing the conversation but with a shade of sadness.*) The film was stupid, Signor, don't you think so?

ALESSANDRO: Absolutely, STUPID AS LIFE ITSELF.

A SPECTATOR: (*Moving off after looking at Angiola with lust, in a low voice.*) Pretty . . . Truly exciting . . .

ALESSANDRO: (*With no conviction.*) Shall we see each other again?

ANGIOLA: Impossible.

MISS JONES: (*Coming out of the theater.*) I should not have stayed until the end of the movie. I missed my train.

ANGIOLA: I have a car.

MOTHER DIDA: (*Muttering, offering her flowers to the people coming out of the theater.*) Fine carnations, beautiful roses . . . Freshly cut, beautiful fresh roses . . .

ALESSANDRO: One minute.

(*He goes to Mother Dida. Angiola lost in thought is putting on her gloves.*)

MOTHER DIDA: Ten lira for the bunch, beautiful roses. Buy the pretty Signora some, Signor.

(*Alessandro buys the roses, gives them to Angiola, kisses her hand.*)

ALESSANDRO: Goodbye, Signora.

(*She slowly exits left. Alessandro takes a few steps to the right.*)

ALESSANDRO: (*To himself.*) Everything is back to normal. Here you are again, in the world where political assassinations are make-believe, where people go to the movies, where women are willing, where you will operate, tomorrow at eight thirty in the morning. Go home . . .

(*A man wearing a Fascist guard's uniform enters quickly from the right, almost running against Alessandro whom he recognizes.*)

THE FASCIST GUARD: It's you? Do you know what happened to you?

ALESSANDRO: What? How? I don't know anything . . . How could I know anything? Tell me, Tommasso.

THE FASCIST GUARD: Your wife . . . Absolutely crazy . . . The Stevo business, I suppose. She waited by the exit of the Palazzo Balbo, by the little door opening on the Piazza San-Giovanni-Martire . . . He was wonderful . . . Calm . . . Your family name . . . Maria . . .

ALESSANDRO: (*Protesting.*) No, not Maria.

THE FASCIST GUARD: How should I know? Marcella Sarte . . . No, she didn't say anything . . . She kept on shooting until . . . Her papers . . . Found on her . . . My poor friend, what a business!

ALESSANDRO: Is she dead? Dead?

THE FASCIST GUARD: Of course she's dead . . . Obviously . . .

ALESSANDRO: (*Controlling himself.*) I see . . . A mad adventure . . . Where did they put her?

THE FASCIST GUARD: Not far from here, at the San Gargano headquarters. You had better go there. There is nothing to fear, Alessandro, I'll vouch for you . . . Your reputation . . .

ALESSANDRO: A mad adventure . . . She dared do THAT. She tried to do THAT.

(They run out. Total darkness.)

SHORT LIT UP SCENE

In what is meant to be the police station, Marcella's body can be seen, lying on a bench, her head thrown back, hanging down. The fringes of the shawl half covering her are dragging on the ground. Alessandro and the policeman are having words with an officer who is gesticulating.

ALESSANDRO: Her name? Sarte, like mine. Born Ardeati. How old? Twenty-nine . . . No, twenty-eight. She lived Via Fosca . . . I recognize her . . . I recognize her . . .

SCENE 2

Piazza Balbo. Mother Dida is sitting between her baskets on the steps of a palace, in front of a Baroque portal adjacent to the Cafe Imperio whose lit up windows can be seen. To the right, one can vaguely make out the front of the Theater Mondo, dark now. The stage is lit both by a street lamp and by the light coming from the cafe.

MOTHER DIDA: (To herself.) Good God Almighty! Everyone bolted because of the storm, and here I am, left all alone, and how could I have made the bus for Ponte-Porzio in this crowd. Now, the last bus for Ponte-Porzio left, and I'm stuck here, soaked to the skin. And the speech, you got to have speeches, but that isn't what sells flowers. For a whole hour, all I saw were the backs of people listening, and the police telling me to move along. How do they want me to move? And these roses, all wilted by the storm, what a shame . . . Of course, when the movie let out, I managed to sell two or three dozen of them. For example, to this man and that pretty girl . . . I bet those two didn't hold themselves back . . . I should have asked him for twenty liras . . . And now, it can't be helped . . . But I won't go spend the night at Attilia's, not before Hell freezes over, no thanks, with all those brats and that bastard Marinunzi. I would wake up, and bye bye my savings, or even worse. (And she pats the little bag that hangs from her neck like a scapular, hidden in her blouse.) And in that street, in that hotel drivers go to, it's too expensive, and not for a good woman like me who owns a house in Ponte-Porzio. I could ask the lady of the cafe to let me sleep in the hall, the hall that leads to the washroom that she lets me use and where I have my water jugs. But mustn't take advantage, otherwise, she won't be willing anymore . . . Pull in your head, under your shawl, Dida, like an old turtle, snuggle in the corner of the step. And tomorrow, Ilario will come with his little flower truck, and I'll have my fresh bunches of flowers. The weather isn't too cold for April, even if the good Lord sees fit to thunder and rain without worrying about people or plants . . . Just pretend that you are young, Mother Dida, that you are spending the night dancing. (*She sinks into deeper and deeper thought.*) Once you were young, and your husband Fruttuoso loved to dance. Until work killed him, of course, a train ran him over because he fell asleep in his cart . . . That was so long ago, that it isn't even sad anymore. Can't say that you couldn't make them work, your men. And all those children . . . Some of them, I don't even know anymore if they're dead or in America. And you're alone, except for all those good for nothings around you, and they don't count. Or rather, you would be alone without your Jesus around your neck, your money, your Sacred Host, the proof that you slaved your whole life long . . . (*The light of the cafe goes out. Sound of an iron gate coming down.*) What's that now? God thundering? No, it's not God, it's the cafe closing. Too late for the washroom. The boss looks all worked up.

(*The owner of the cafe is bolting the iron gate noisily, then turns towards Dida. She seems all excited and happy to be so.*)

THE LADY OF THE CAFE: Dida, hey, Dida!

DIDA: I'm not doing anything wrong, Signora Erminia. I'm here because I missed the eleven ten bus, the one that goes to Ponte-Porzio. And I'm too old to be sleeping out; if at least I could be out of the rain in a hall . . .

THE LADY OF THE CAFE: (*Screaming at the top of her lungs.*) Forget your bus. Someone shot Him, Dida! You don't know anything, you're sitting there like a stump . . . We are living in terrible times! A customer told me . . .

DIDA: Of course it's not the right weather for the time of year, Signora Erminia.

THE LADY OF THE CAFE: (*In the same voice.*) What? I'm telling you someone tried to shoot Him as he was leaving, on the little piazza, on the other side of Palazzo Balbo. A customer saw the mark of the bullets on the car window . . . It just missed . . . It was a woman, imagine that . . . and young, it seems. Another attempt by these know-nothing anarchists, socialists, communists, who knows what, those people who get money from abroad . . . We've been too soft on them, Mother Dida . . . And the woman? Dead, of course . . . They had to . . . She fought, she hung on . . . Some say they were grenades, not bullets . . . It seems that there is blood on the ground at the entrance to San-Giovanni-Martire . . . A puddle of blood . . . Goodnight, Dida, I'm sure I won't sleep a wink tonight. (*She leaves.*)

DIDA: (*To herself, thoughtfully.*) Well, it's like the time someone shot the King, the year Ilario was born. (*She huddles down among her baskets.*) How dark it is, really . . . the owner left, she doesn't care what becomes of me without that bus; she has other things on her mind, of course . . . How big the piazza is when there is no one there . . . So they shot at the man that the King said should rule . . . It's not a world for Christians and even beasts would know better . . . and He saved the country, for sure, even if things haven't changed at Ponte-Porzio . . . It's true that He's hard on those who are against him: the other day, the Menotti son was put in prison; it was sad . . . And those who protest, they make them drink castor-oil; that's dirty. And everything costs more, can't deny it . . . Still, it's a crime . . . A puddle of blood . . . She must have had courage to do such a thing, that woman. Maybe they had hurt her in some way . . . In the name of the Father, in the name of the Son . . . It can't be a sin to say a little prayer for her . . . And who knows, maybe sooner than you think, Dida, you will be glad to have someone do the same thing for you. (*She crosses herself, then looks around her furtively, worriedly.*) What if there was someone still hovering at the back of the piazza, in front of San-Giovanni-Martire . . . No, no one . . . It's just the police, as always, walking side by side . . . Yes, and they already sprinkled the blood with sand. Yet, Death passed by there; it didn't take Him, but it took the woman; perhaps it is still roaming around, looking for someone else . . . When the time comes, there's nothing you can do. And what came over the damn priest this morning to say that I would be resurrected fist clenched? (*She lifts her hand up to her face, opens it and moves her fingers.*) Am I stingy? What does it mean to be stingy? I will tell you, little priest, it's to know that you are poor. In this stinking world, where no one helps you . . . So I gave the good Lord nothing? The churches are packed with gods; they are born at Christmas; they die at Easter; they aren't concerned with people. And Tullia and Maria, my wretched daughters, why should I give them money? They are just bright enough to scratch the ground; you don't need new skirts for that. And Ilario, it's only right that he work for nothing since he will inherit some day . . . And if I don't want him to marry, it's because girls today are worthless . . . Is it my fault that Attilia married a bum who drinks and vomits what she makes? And what can I do if Luca, Maria's father, the workman I took when I needed someone, me, poor widow, now drags himself along the road—an old beggar who will be found someday, dead as a mule, in a field. He's no longer of any use; what would people say in Ponte-Porzio if I had kept him eating off the family? And one of these days, that bastard Marinunzi will be waiting for me at the bus stop, on that stretch of road, and because of my little bag, he'll cut my throat with his knife . . . Or Ilario will fix it so that it will look like an accident . . . Old women are known to fall in wells . . . Ah yes, of course, God who thunders . . . The weather is clearing up, but there is still some lightning, especially toward Ponte-Porzio . . . Maybe at this very moment, a beggar is sneaking into the greenhouse with a lighter; he is setting a fire, but people will think that lightning struck. At Judgment Day, God will burn the weeds. (*She suddenly snaps out of her reverie and notices Clément Roux who appears at the corner of the piazza. He is weary, soaked, his hat drawn over his eyes; he looks like a poor man.*) And what is this old man doing here, all alone, at this hour? No, he's not one of those dirty bums who steal and light fires. He looks honest; he is a good poor man . . . Come to think of it, on such a night, it's reassuring to see someone alive here . . . He is soaked through; he must have roamed around all night long. Maybe he's like me and doesn't know where to go to sleep. You never gave anything away, Mother Dida, not even a bone to a dog. What if I gave him this new coin; that couldn't do any harm; he's not from the neighborhood; he won't come back to ask . . . And furthermore, who knows? He looks like the Good Lord fallen into poverty . . . And when the day comes, they won't be able to say anymore that Dida is close-fisted. (*She draws the ten lira piece out of her pocket and offers it to Clément Roux.*) Here, old man. For you.

CLÉMENT ROUX: (*Startled, turning the coin around in his hand.*) Well, I must say . . . It's the first time something like that happened to me. (*He exits slowly.*)

DIDA: It was too much for him; it really gave him a shock. I should have given him only one lira. Well, so that's all there is to it. I really shut him up, little Father Cicca. And now what? The weather is clearing up, for sure; the concierge of the Conti Palazzo will let me sleep in his courtyard. And if I put these flowers in water, tomorrow I'm bound to be able to palm them off on someone. Mustn't look at the dark side of things, Mother Dida. (*She leaves.*)

SCENE 3

Streets of Rome. The stage has only three props that will be lit in turn as needed. When the curtain rises, we see on the left side, towards the back of the stage, a balustrade overhanging what is meant to be ruins from the Forum, and a stone bench near a fragment of a column of classical times; towards center stage, a wall with Fascist graffiti. Clément Roux will lean against the foot of this wall for a few moments; at the very right of the stage, towards the footlights, a fountain with a very low brink, and perhaps a Baroque statue, Neptune, or Triton, or a sea horse. The slow and sinuous walk of Clément Roux and Massimo, often interrupted and followed by a spotlight, will take place between these three spots; it is meant to be a walk in the imaginary streets of Rome. Clément Roux is leaning on the balustrade now, on the right. The stage is lit by a moonlight light.

CLÉMENT ROUX: It's no longer so beautiful; the ruins are too tidy. Too demolished, too reconstructed. In my day, these little streets zigzagged, and led you to the monuments by surprise. All that has been replaced by magnificent thoroughfares for buses or, should the occasion arise, for tanks . . .. Haussmann's Paris. The fairground of ruins, Permanent Exhibition of the Roman World. *Laudator temporis acti?* No, it's ugly. And in any case, too tiresome . . . This pain is really too . . . (*He leans harder on the balustrade.*) The vise is tightening . . . What is going to happen to me this time? Calm yourself, try to deflect the crisis one more time. Doctor Sarte's prescription is in my left pocket. (*He gropes in his pocket, pulls out a glass tube, breaks it, inhales deeply.*)

(*Massimo, standing at the edge of the shadows on the left, observes him.*)

MASSIMO: (*In a soft voice.*) Do you need anything?
CLÉMENT ROUX: (*Snapping.*) Selling postcards?
MASSIMO: Don't be afraid. I'm not selling anything tonight. Problems with the heart?

(*He holds Clément Roux up, almost forcing him to sit down on the bench. For a while, neither of them speaks.*)

CLÉMENT ROUX: (*Catching his breath.*) Hell, I'm done for.
MASSIMO: (*His back leaning against the balustrade, in a soft voice, lighting a cigarette.*) No, Monsieur Roux, not yet. On the contrary, you are feeling better.
CLÉMENT ROUX: (*Disturbed, to himself.*) What? . . . I can hardly hear him. Where did he come from? Pale, looks like he just pulled off something, something bad. His hands are shaking . . . It doesn't matter; it's good that he's here . . . (*Holding his hand out towards Massimo's cigarettes.*) Give me one.
MASSIMO: No. It's not good for you.
CLÉMENT ROUX: (*Humbly.*) That's true. But I feel better. In fact, much better, because you know, the false alarms . . . Tired of dying, tired of not dying, tired of everything. But you couldn't understand. How old are you?
MASSIMO: Twenty-two.
CLÉMENT ROUX: That's what I thought. I'm seventy . . .
MASSIMO: (*To himself.*) Twenty-two . . . And she's been dead for a hundred years now, and Carlo, for ten centuries . . . Dead. Vanished . . . This woman I could hear breathing next to me, her hand in my hand. And him with his gasping breath, and his suit we took to a Viennese tailor to be mended, his passion for German music . . . A sum whisked off that total. INCONCEIVABLE. This old man recovering from his heart pain doesn't know that he's solid ground for me, someone alive . . .
CLÉMENT ROUX: It's been thirty years since I last saw Rome. Changed for the worst, uglier, like everything else. Oh, I guess that a young lad, like yourself, finds in this a sort of beauty you too will miss in thirty years. Not for me anymore . . . I hate noise; I despise crowds. But nevertheless, tonight I couldn't stand it in the reception rooms of their Caesar Palace . . . So I went

on, all alone, on foot . . .

MASSIMO: (*In a strangled voice.*) Like everyone else. To hear a speech in Piazza Balbo.

CLÉMENT ROUX: Not on your life! Go watch people bray acclamations to a howling man? You don't know me, my friend. No, but dark streets. Deserted. Precisely because the crowd poured out on one side like a pail being emptied. And the angry rain on the buildings . . . And me under an arch of the Coliseum, smoking, left in peace. Then a little lost in these changed streets . . . But the funniest thing is that not everything disappears at the same speed. There are certain corners, balconies, doors, things I didn't remember and that I remembered nevertheless since when I saw them I recognized them. And then putting my feet down on the pavement a little more carefully than before, you see, and feeling its unevenness more, its wear and tear. Am I boring you?

MASSIMO: You're not boring me in the least, Monsieur Roux. I am thinking about a small painting of yours, an early one, which shows a corner of Rome, a landscape of very human ruins . . . Even considering everything you've done since then, it's still very beautiful. Or was already very beautiful.

CLÉMENT ROUX: (*Suspiciously.*) You know who I am?

MASSIMO: It's very simple: the other day I saw your self-portrait at the Triennial Exhibition of Modern Art. (*To himself.*) I'm getting used to it. I'm already used enough to their death to be able to talk about painting. And besides, I'm flattering him. I only recognized him because of the newspaper pictures. Poor great man . . . A little admiration will do him good.

CLÉMENT ROUX: (*In his same muttering tone, thoughtfully.*) Well then, you know an old fool. Clément Roux, all kidding aside. You're French? No, Russian, I recognized the accent. Me, I'm from Hazebrouck. Because you got to be from somewhere. The portrait isn't bad; you have taste. Portraits, no one does them anymore, because people don't give a damn about human beings. And because it's too difficult. You have to take a face, pull it apart, put it back together, add up a series of spontaneous moments . . . Not your face; you're too handsome. It's not worth it. But a mug like mine. Your landscape of very human ruins, you might say. You are lucky to be twenty-two.

MASSIMO: (*To himself, looking away.*) Luck . . . Talk about luck. To be the one who doesn't die, the one who watches, the one who never quite enters the game completely. To be the one who tries to save, or on the contrary . . . The Angel of the last hours . . . And Marcella's look, I'll never forget it . . . I can't help it if they love me. That hour stolen from time at the end of everything . . . And I found nothing better to do than getting drunk on words . . . In order to encourage her, to hold her back? . . . Yes. But mostly to hide that their world wasn't mine. The real betrayal was not to have yielded to that agent's blackmail in Vienna, during that business with the passports . . . Even less, this obligatory visit last fall to that bogus character whose desk in Palazzo Vedoni had all those pigeonholes . . . No, you like the illicit . . . No, don't defend yourself; don't turn the thing into a gloomy joke. My name is somewhere on their lists. Contaminated forever as by syphilis or leprosy. Live on, for forty years, with festering symptoms of a forgiven infamy. Tomorrow, I'll be summoned again by the bogus character; I'll be asked questions that I'll answer once again with the opposite of the truth. They're not so dumb, only half dumb. They'll judge me incompetent or an accomplice. And, considering my status as a foreigner, they'll ask me to leave their lovely Italy, and to have my make-shift passport stamped elsewhere . . . Once again, my filthy luck . . . It will all boil down to a visit to my mother, who sells antiques in Vienna.

(*Clément Roux, who for a moment dozed off, head against the back of the bench, wakes up and is now observing Massimo attentively during the last few lines of his speech.*)

CLÉMENT ROUX: What is the matter with you? You look like you're crying.

MASSIMO: (*Savagely.*) No, I'm not crying. I don't even have the right. (*After a pause.*) A young woman was killed tonight. After the speech. It wasn't an accident. An attempted political assassination on her part.

CLÉMENT ROUX: Where?

MASSIMO: Not far from here. On the little piazza of San-Giovanni-Martire.

CLÉMENT ROUX: (*With respect.*) Poor wench!

MASSIMO: (*To himself.*) I shouldn't have told him that. He's too old and sick to worry about other people's misfortune.

CLÉMENT ROUX: (*To himself, rising, with a shade of anxiety in his voice.*) This remission won't last. Might as well take advantage of it to go home. Get away from here . . . And tomorrow leave Rome.

MASSIMO: A taxi?

CLÉMENT ROUX: Not right away . . . First I'd like . . . And besides, there aren't any. (*To himself.*) And expensive this late at night. If this slightly shady but obliging youth would be willing to accompany me . . . I still have at least one vial on me. After all, it's probably nothing more than a false alarm.

MASSIMO: Are you sure you can walk?

CLÉMENT ROUX: A little. It's rather good for me. It's not that far. Let's go by Piazza Santi Apostoli.

MASSIMO: He's proud that he knows Rome so well.

(*They take a few steps.*)

CLÉMENT ROUX: That woman? Were you there?

MASSIMO: (*Violently.*) No! No!

CLÉMENT ROUX: And Him? Is He unhurt?

MASSIMO: (*Bitterly.*) Not a scratch. People say she missed by a hair.

CLÉMENT ROUX: What damned luck! Oh, of course, sooner or later, his luck will run out. The risks of the job. In my youth, there was a popular refrain of Bruant about some sort of underworld thug: *He croaked like a Caesar . . .* That's it: croaked like a Caesar. I'm not saying that to belittle Him, on the contrary . . . Somebody's got to run things, since most people are too soft to do the job. And you know, me and politics . . . And besides, I'm not from here . . . Only as long as he doesn't lead us to war.

MASSIMO: (*With conviction.*) Precisely. I'm not from here either.

CLÉMENT ROUX: (*Starting to walk again.*) I'll tell you what they make me think of, your politics. I have a friend who's director of the orchestra at La Scala. He told me that when they need crowd noises, the sounds of riot, people howling for or against, what have you, they get deep voices to sing from the wings one single beautiful, highly sonorous word: RUBARBARA. In rounds . . . BARBARARU . . . BARARUBAR . . . RARUBARBA. See what I mean. Well, politics, whether of the left or the right, it's rhubarb to me, my boy.

MASSIMO: (*Hesitating.*) Monsieur Clément Roux, you were in the 1914 war. How did you get used to knowing that the comrades you lived with would perhaps in an hour, almost without fail . . . That woman, for example. Well, she was a member of the same group . . . The friend of a friend. (*To himself.*) Of a friend? The rest counted so little for me. And for him? A clandestine passerby whom you turn into a disciple for want of anything better . . . A means to regain a certain moment of his youth . . . A reaction against his leftist puritanism. And if it counted for more than that, it was in a realm words don't enter. (*To Clément Roux.*) A friend. But I had introduced myself under false pretenses. (*To himself.*) No, that is not quite the truth either. From Kitzbuhel on, I warned him; I even advised him never to come back to Italy. I couldn't do anymore . . . But from that time on, for him, the die was cast. (*To Clément Roux.*) A dead friend. And that woman, I followed her from afar a while back, cautiously . . . I learned about it by chance, at the entrance of a cafe, at a respectable distance from it all, as they say. Oh, I was free not to believe in the effectiveness of political assassination! All the same, she must have despised me as she died. (*He turns his head away as if to hide tears.*)

CLÉMENT ROUX: (*Alarmed, to himself.*) What's he going on about? (*To Massimo*) Well, my boy, I don't understand a word of your story. First of all, to begin with, where are you from? The gentleman conspires? No? So much the better. Do you have a family? No, right? An address?

MASSIMO: Until tomorrow morning.

CLÉMENT ROUX: I thought as much. And how do you make a living?

MASSIMO: (*Bitter.*) I deal in false passports.

CLÉMENT ROUX: Ah! Well then, my friend, you're out of luck with me. Even if I didn't have one in my pocket. Don't feel like going anywhere anymore. Unless you have one good enough to get me through Heaven's Gates.

MASSIMO: (*Seriously.*) You mustn't say that, Monsieur Roux.

(*Clement Roux stops, leans against a wall whose top is smeared with politics graffiti of the times, traced in large, uneven letters so that it appears to have been done spontaneously by people walking by:* VV IL . . . VIVERE PERICOLOSAMENTE . . . AVANTI . . . PER NON DORMIRE . . . VV L'IMPERO . . . PERICOL . . .)

CLÉMENT ROUX: (*Dreamingly, to himself.*) This street, I'll probably never come here again . . . And this Rome. I should look around me . . . All the more because it is, after all, really beautiful . . . Especially by this clean night, washed by the storm; this night almost not of this world . . . The almost imperceptible curves of these buildings rounding off space . . . Moreover, I feel fine . . . Surprisingly fine . . . Yet, walking as if I had the brake on. If something happened, this boy could always get help . . . Unless . . . The newspaper headlines tomorrow: Clément Roux found dead of a heart attack in the street, mugged by . . . No, not dangerous, unhappy, slightly mythomaniac perhaps. If a taxi comes by, it would be a good idea to flag it down.

MASSIMO: (*With weariness, to himself.*) If a taxi comes by, it would be prudent to have him take it. The last one was full.

CLÉMENT ROUX: (*Starting to walk again.*) Speaking of the war of '14, at that time I was already too old . . . My brother is the one who got himself killed at Craonne. But they lied about it so much that even those who came back no longer know. And not only about the war, but about life . . . So, when the Italian reporters ask me about myself . . . My mother, she wanted me to be a priest. Picture her, the lady of the farm in her plush hat she wore only for high mass. And then Paris, and work, and the usual lousy problems of the artist not making it. And then, fame . . . For no reason, because the wind shifted. I never realized that there were that many art dealers in the world, people who speculate on art. The Stock Exchange, the Outside Bettors, what have you. And those who used me to knock down the great ones of the previous day, who said that Renoir was no big deal, that Manet was warm beer . . . Then the time comes when you are so well known that nobody cares anymore: Clément Roux, classified. And in ten years, people will stick the paintings in their attics because they'll be out of fashion; and in fifty years they'll hang in museums again, even those that are forgeries, and, in two hundred years, people will say that Clément Roux never existed, that it was really someone else, or that there were several Roux . . . My fame . . . Where was I? My memories. My wife, an excellent woman, the best of women. Good housekeeper, not even jealous. And pretty at the beginning, the whitest body imaginable: like milk. Of course, you know her, I painted her. Two years of love, a child with a little white collar in the paintings of 1905, and who now sells cars, and another who is dead. And the lady growing old, losing weight, becoming difficult (always the proper lady, you know); you no longer feel like making love to her, no more than you would to a church-club matron . . . Yes, I also painted her in that mode, in a gray dress. And then, she died. What a change! And you get used to it . . . And you get used to not getting used to it. And your countrywoman, Sabine Bagration, who takes it into her head to love me, and moves me into her villa on the Riviera, and then threatens me with her gun . . . A slim woman, not beautiful, but interesting. A woman who loved unhappiness, like you. And she had plenty of it; in her country, she got herself thrown down a mine shaft . . . And then what else? All in all, I didn't live that much . . . Painting takes a lot of discipline. You have to get up early . . Go to bed early . . . I don't have any memories.

MASSIMO: (*To himself.*) And that is what this illustrious old fool got out of his life . . . Of course, there are always his masterpieces . . . And you, where will you be at his age? Or even in ten years? A hotel clerk? A correspondent for an evening newspaper? An aging Narcissus who looks into shop windows to see if adventure will come his way? . . . Or perhaps a fanatic passing out pamphlets about the coming of the Lord? . . . Don't worry . . . Wait. Accept even the fact that you did not want her; you loved her more than you ever loved any woman, but couldn't stand the oily, spicy smell of her hair . . . Accept not having quite believed in what they did . . . Accept the fact that they are dead; you too will die one day. Wait . . . Start from what you are . . . Right now, you are escorting back to his hotel this pitiful great man in an artsy costume of 1900. Out of loyalty to the style of his youth? How sentimental! These French peoples . . .

CLÉMENT ROUX: (*Stopping, a little lost.*) Where are we?

MASSIMO: Humility Street, Monsieur Clément Roux, Via del l'Umilità. (*Neither speaks for a while, they keep on walking then.*) By the way, Monsieur Roux, I wanted to tell you . . . This dead friend . . . This Carlo Stevo.

CLÉMENT ROUX: (*Absentmindedly.*) Yes, I know who Carlo Stevo is.

MASSIMO: (*In a shaking voice, opening himself up all the more easily because he no longer hopes to be listened to.*) I know this can't really interest you, but still, it's a little like your memories. No one understands. And oblivion comes so quickly. Oh, they talk about Carlo Stevo; they'll talk about him even more tomorrow when they find out he's dead. But without knowing . . . Those not insulting him will call him a great writer, a genius sidetracked by politics . . . All this noise about a wretched, extorted letter, but no one, not even me, dares to envisage brutalities, physical suffering, weariness, doubts at the moment of death . . . No, no one. And they can't understand that a dying man is willing to look as if yielding, as if giving up what he thought he believed in, that he might want to die alone, even without convictions, all alone . . . Carlo Stevo and his courage to go all the way in everything, to the limits of his strength, beyond that strength . . . To succumb with shame, to be ridiculed . . . To speak German badly, for example . . . His capacity to understand, his incapacity to despise . . . His wonderful feeling for Beethoven; those evenings in the room in Spiegelgasse when we played all the records of the last quartets . . . His sad man's cheerfulness . . . And his books everyone talks about but no longer reads. And in the long run, I'm the only one left as witness . . . Had he lived, perhaps I would have learned something . . . (*He recites the prayer for the dead in ecclesiastic Old Slavonic, in a low voice.*) TZARSTVO TEBE NEBESNOE . . .

CLÉMENT ROUX: (*Continuing his own thoughts.*) All that . . . Well . . . Well . . .

(*They both stop near the basin of a fountain.*)

CLÉMENT ROUX: (*Enchanted.*) The fountain with the Tritons . . . My god, how beautiful! Help me down the step. It's very slippery. I would like to sit for a while on the rim. (*He sits down.*)

MASSIMO: (*Standing, to himself.*) Water that washes, water one drinks, water that loses and assumes all forms. Water that was perhaps denied someone suffering from fever on Lipari Island . . .

CLÉMENT ROUX: (*Garrulous, a little senile.*) You see, I wouldn't want you to think that . . . There are some worthwhile things . . . This fountain, for example, I wanted to see it again before leaving, but in this damn city, you never know what you will be able to find again . . . Things so beautiful that you're surprised that they are still there. Bits, fragments . . . Paris, gray all over, Rome, golden . . . That column, over there, where we were, did you see it, like the needle of a moon dial? And the Coliseum, that is really something, isn't it, a well-baked pate with a thick stone crust, stuffed with gladiators inside. And then everywhere, anything, a coffeepot or a cathedral . . . And wonderful faces, like yours . . . and then, bodies . . . (*After a pause.*) Women's bodies . . . Not models, nude for so much per hour . . . Nor the nakedness of whores, nor of burlesque covered with so much make-up you can no longer see the skin . . . And almost never a perfect foot among them, firm and pure . . . But from time to time . . . A bit of flesh under the garment, like a sweet secret in this hard world. The body behind the clothing . . . The soul behind the body . . . The soul of the body . . . Once, a long time ago, on a deserted beach in Sicily, a little naked girl . . . Twelve or thirteen . . . In the faint daylight of early morning . . . Innocent and not innocent . . . you see, the young Venus emerging from the sea . . . And her legs a little paler than the rest of her because you saw them underwater. Oh, don't go thinking: no, too young, and furthermore, too beautiful . . . Even though I could have, after all . . . And I didn't paint her either, because nudes painted from memory . . . But I put her here and there, everywhere, in a certain way of showing light playing on a body. These are things that help when your time to die has come. (*He pulls up the collar of his cloak.*) I think . . . I think that I'm catching cold.

MASSIMO: You have to go home, Monsieur Clément Roux. It's after one o'clock.

CLÉMENT ROUX: (*Half rambling.*) Yes, I understand. Closing time, gentlemen . . . Don't be impatient. First I must finish Baroness Bernheim's portrait. I'm going back to France. Doctor Sarte says that this country is not good for me this time of year. The first hot spells. I hope that the valet secured my trunk firmly. The ten-fifteen train . . . (*He is compulsively squeezing Massimo's fingers. In a confidential tone.*) It's hard to leave when you're beginning to understand, when you've learned. And one keeps on painting, adding forms to this world full of forms . . . In spite of fatigue. I used to be in strapping health, you know, like a farmhand . . . And even today, on the days I feel well, I feel eternal. Only, when things go wrong, there is now someone in me who says yes. Says yes to death . . . (*He takes a coin out of his pocket and turns it over in the palm of his hand.*) During the rain shower, as I told you, I took cover under an arch. Soaked, even so. An old woman must have taken me for a beggar. She gave me this. Isn't that funny? Oh, don't misunderstand me; she wasn't drunk. Maybe it was a restitution.

MASSIMO: (*To himself.*) He's the one who is drunk. Drunk with fatigue . . . This grotesque, this pitiful funeral vigil.

CLÉMENT ROUX: And those travelers leaving, if they throw a coin in the water it is said that they'll come back. As for me, for what I would be doing here, in Rome, I'm not tempted to come back. Rather see something else, something really new, with fresh eyes, eyes washed pure . . . But what else is there? Who's really seen the Eternal City? Life, my friend, might only begin on the day after the Resurrection.

MASSIMO: Well, Monsieur Roux, are you coming?

CLÉMENT ROUX: (*Solemnly.*) Yes. (*He throws the coin awkwardly in the basin of the fountain.*)

MASSIMO: (*Ironically.*) It would have been better to give it to me.

CLÉMENT ROUX: You want my money?

MASSIMO: (*Firmly.*) I want to take you home. I can't leave you stranded at the water's edge.

(*Clément Roux rises painfully, gripping Massimo's arm, and stumbles. Massimo helps him to sit down again on the rim of the fountain.*)

CLÉMENT ROUX: (*Terrified.*) I'm not feeling well . . . Wait a minute.

MASSIMO: (*Worried.*) I'll go get you a taxi. Piazza Colonna is just around the corner.

CLÉMENT ROUX: (*Terrified.*) Don't leave me alone! (*Massimo leaves quickly. To*

himself.) He left me alone. To drop dead in this opera setting . . . No one . . .
What if I screamed, that worker repairing something over there wouldn't
hear me. The noise of the water running . . .

(*Sound of the taxi braking, stopping. In its headlights, Massimo can be seen appearing
again, followed by the taxi driver.*)

MASSIMO: I found you a taxi, Monsieur Roux. (*He helps him to get up and directs
him towards the car.*)
THE DRIVER: (*Approaching to help.*) Where to?
MASSIMO: (*To Clément Roux.*) To Caesar Palace, right? (*Clément Roux shakes
his head yes. To the driver.*) To Caesar Palace.

(*Clément Roux disappears, held up by the driver. Massimo moves backwards, raises
his hand to wave goodbye, lit up fully by the headlights of the car.*)

CLÉMENT ROUX'S VOICE: (*Coming from the wings, indistinctively.*) I really should
have asked him for his name.

(*The taxi takes off. The headlights turn and disappear. Total darkness.*)

SCENE 4

*Rome at night. The stage is dark through this scene. Lights will briefly flash on corners
or on moveable platforms whereupon will appear the characters of these little lit-up
scenes with a minimum of props and sets. On the stage itself, nothing but the rim of
the fountain that appeared already in the previous scene and that alone will be visible
at the end of this act.*

VOICE OF THE POET: (*Cold, distant.*) It is dark on the plains, in the hills, dark in
the city, dark on the sea. In the museums of Rome, night fills the rooms that
house the masterpieces: *The Sleeping Fury, The Hermaphrodite, Venus, The
Wounded Gladiator*; marble blocks submit to the great laws that rule the
equilibrium, the weight, the density, the dilation, and the contraction of
stones, unaware of the fact that artisans, dead for thousands of years,
fashioned their surface to the image of creatures of another realm. The ruins
of ancient monuments are of a piece with the night, privileged fragments, of
the past, safe behind their gate, with the ticket taker's empty chair next to
the entrance turnstile. At the Triennial Exhibition of Modern Art, the paintings are now only rectangles of canvas mounted on frames, unevenly caked
with layers of colors that right now are black. On the slopes of the Capitol,
in her lair behind bars, the wolf howls at the night; protected from humans,

but still made uneasy by their proximity, she shudders at the rumble of a few trucks driving by the hill. It is the hour when, in stables attached to slaughterhouses, the beasts, who tomorrow will wind up on dinner plates and in the sewers of Rome, are chewing on a mouthful of straw, and lean their soft and sleepy muzzles on the necks of their fettered companions. It's the hour when in the hospitals the sick who cannot sleep lie impatiently waiting for the next round of the nurse; it's the hour when the girls in the brothel sitting-room tell themselves that soon they'll be able to go to sleep. In newspaper printshops, the presses are turning, grinding out for the morning readers a re-arranged version of yesterday's events; true or false, news crackles in telephone receivers; gleaming rails trace patterns of departure in the dark. (*The voice of the poet is accompanied by nocturnal indistinctive sounds during his recitation, the constant passage of trucks; now and then a train whistle.*) From the top to the bottom of dark houses, sleepers are stacked like the dead along the walls of catacombs; spouses sleep bearing in their damp and warm bodies the living beings of the future: the rebels, the resigned, the violent, the swindlers, the saints, the fools, the martyrs. The song of the fountains rises purer and clearer in the silence of the night. A vegetal darkness, swollen with sap and breezes, unfolds and shudders in the pine trees of Villa Borghese. Clément Roux is sleeping in the middle of a still-life of yawning suitcases, shoes strewn anywhere, sweaters hanging from armchairs. He is feeling better; he sleeps avidly; his body is a mass of gray flesh and gray hair. In the next room, the night is wrapped softly around a sleeping Angiola Fides. In her bathroom, Alessandro's roses are lying in a basin of water. Dida sleeps like a hen between her two baskets in the courtyard of the Palazzo Conti. Caesar is asleep, forgetting he is Caesar. He wakes up, slips on his personage, his fame, lights his lamp for a moment, looks at his wristwatch to tell the time . . .

(*In the back of the stage, to the right, the light shines on a platform where there is a heavily gilded chair upon which have been carefully placed the black shirt of the Dictator, his belt, his black head-dress. In front of the chair are his boots. A huge bed, only half seen, is also heavily gilded, and stands somewhat in the shadows.*)

VOICE OF THE DICTATOR: Must not let the foreign press get hold of this story and exaggerate it . . . But this attempt will serve to enforce stricter measures. Ardeati, née Ardeati . . . Old Giacomo's daughter . . . The smoky kitchen in Cesena where mother Ardeati served coffee while her man and I discussed the comparative merits of Marx and Engels. In those days, coffee seemed a great treat . . . Not a bad woman, Mother Ardeati . . . I've amalgamated into my program what was best in those kinds of minds. You have to kick people around to make them into a great nation . . . Those windbags would never have been able to rule the country. (*The light goes out. We can tell by his voice that he is falling asleep again.*) Ardeati, née Ardeati . . . I have shown the composure befitting a statesman. The recent visit of General Goering and of Colonel Von Papen. I have the approval of law and order citizens.

THE VOICE OF THE POET: Giulio Lovisi is not sleeping. He is going over his accounts.

(*In the back, the light shines on a sort of nook showing Giulio Lovisi in his armchair, pencil and book in hand. Giovanna is standing near him; she is wearing a robe. There is a door behind them.*)

GIULIO LOVISI: *Chanel Number Two*, three dozens. *Evening in Paris*, five and a half. *China Crepe* . . . (*To Giovanna.*) You better go to sleep.

GIOVANNA: I can't sleep, Daddy. How much do you think we'll need now that everything is going to be all right? Our old apartment in Parioli is still vacant. I could tell the manager that by the end of May . . . But first, we'll go rest on a real beach.

GIULIO LOVISI: Not so fast, my daughter. These formalities take a lot of time. And really, your plans aren't . . . Don't forget that your husband is a sick man.

GIOVANNA: Precisely. Maybe they'll allow him to go to Switzerland to see a doctor. (*Thinking.*) I'll have to have my summer suit mended.

GIUSEPPA: (*Very angry, sticking her head through the slight opening of the door.*) Be quiet! You are going to wake up the child!

(*The light goes out. They disappear.*)

THE VOICE OF THE POET: Alessandro is not sleeping either. He is being detained at police headquarters.

(*The light now shows at the back of the stage Alessandro and a high official sitting across a wide, ministerial type of desk. On this desk, a tray with a carafe and glasses. Alessandro seems worn out but in perfect control of himself. The official is courteous but firm. He is wearing a costume decorated with many medals which he probably wore at the reception at Palazzo Balbo.*)

THE OFFICIAL: Your reputation is not threatened, Doctor Sarte. You are one of us. A glass of water? . . . But you arrived at your wife's towards seven o'clock; you left around eight o'clock. It is difficult to see how . . .

ALESSANDRO: (*With a controlled irritation.*) I see, Excellency, I'll have to explain the whole thing once again. In 1928, my wife . . .

(*The light goes out. They disappear.*)

THE VOICE OF THE POET: Father Cicca goes down the steps of his building, and heads towards the church for early mass.

(*A pale gray light accompanies Father Cicca as he crosses the stage. Faint sound of bells.*)

FATHER CICCA: Lord, my eyes are open on You, as soon as morning comes . . . Today is a day that the Lord created . . . This morning You will hear my prayer . . .

(*He disappears. The gray light stays.*)

VOICE OF THE POET: The dead are asleep but no one knows their dreams. Lina Chiari is sleeping with her cancer. She is thinking about Massimo who is not thinking about her.

LINA'S VOICE: (*Faintly.*) He did promise he would call tomorrow morning. Sleep in peace, my girl . . . O God, see to it that I fall asleep.

(*On the left of the stage, the light now shines on a platform that is to be taken as Massimo's room. There is a bed, a small table on which there is an open suitcase, a stool with books. A suit, carefully placed on a coat hanger, hangs from a coat rack. Half dressed, lying across his bed, Massimo is sleeping. A naked lightbulb hanging from the ceiling is on.*)

MASSIMO: (*Waking up with a start, still at the border of unconsciousness.*) Lots of snow . . . What was under all that snow? . . . A van in the middle of fir woods . . . You are dreaming; wake up . . . (*He sits up at the edge of the bed. After a while, he suddenly covers his face with his elbow as if someone were going to hit him.*) And it's already yesterday that they died . . . (*He rises, turns out the light. A weak gray light invades the stage. Bitterly.*) The dawn of a fine day. (*A pause. He stays stock still as though nailed to the bed.*) Dead? . . . Set. Unalterable. Indestructible. And you will change; you will forget them, or you will think you have forgotten them, or maybe you will remember, but what you were for them, or them for you, that will never change now. Set forever. And now? . . . (*He takes his suit off the rack.*) This suit is almost new . . . It's a good thing I had Duetti make it for me before leaving Rome . . . (*Interrupting himself, disgusted.*) Ah, your frivolity is almost obscene . . . First pack your books. (*He goes up to the shelf and looks at his books.*) You will never be able to take all that . . . Kierkegaard . . . I read it; that's enough. Berdiaeff, Chestov, someday I'll buy them again. Apollinaire . . . (*He opens the book and reads.*)

Un soir de demi-brume à Londres,
Un voyou qui ressemblait à
Mon amour vint à ma rencontre . . .

Enough. (*He puts the book down again, picks up another.*) Rilke: "God, give each of us his own death . . ." Poems that one likes can be remembered without books. Carlo Stevo . . . (*His fingers touch one or two books lightly, then he takes one. He reads to himself for a while.*) Still, I should take something from him. (*He slips that book in his suitcase, closes the lid, then sits down at the table and puts his elbows on it.*) That book will travel with me. I am sleepy. (*His head begins to nod. Already dreaming.*) Naked bodies in the snow. Heaps of them on the snow. (*Half conscious still.*) I can still sleep a little. Morning hasn't broken yet.

(*He falls asleep, his head between his hands. He disappears. A bottle in each hand, Marinunzi comes in from the right towards the rim of the fountain. The light of dawn invades the stage.*)

MARINUNZI: Looks like there aren't as many tourists in Rome these days, or else they've all gone broke . . . People say that in the old days, they used to throw gold in the fountain. Just the same, with what I fished out in dunking myself . . . And I know a good place, near the train station, that is only closed for fools; you can't buy a drink, because it isn't open, but you can buy something to drink because it's not closed. I got every right to sit down here among the tools of my trade. (*He sits down on the ground. With melancholy.*) Drink, Oreste, it's better than to go home. Besides, what would I do now if I went home? When I left to fix this leak, Attilia's hair was untied, because it's easier that way; and the neighbor to the right was boiling water; and the old lady from across the hall was warming up soup, and Attilia was crying even though she is used to giving birth . . . What a mess! And it is only right to let the women manage among themselves . . . To the health of number five! (*He gets up, drinks in turn from both bottles. In a confidential tone.*) After all, Attilia and me could get along without number five, but when they come, what can you do? . . . It's that sneaky Ilario's fault; if Mother Dida had a heart, number five would bring in money instead of costing us; we could get our wardrobe back from the pawn shop . . . Drink to Mother Dida's health, Oreste, because if she drops dead, she won't even leave you enough for you and Attilia to buy mourning clothes . . . Those people don't appreciate me . . . Just because one day I said that it would be nice to strangle the old lady, that shifty Ilario treats me like a murderer, me who wouldn't hurt a fly . . . And yet, it's true that it would do us all good if one day, at the bus stop, on that lonely road where no one would hear her squawk . . . And that little bag she wears around her neck, no one would be the wiser . . . After all, it belongs to Attilia, it's only fair . . . But those things are risky; nothing's more treacherous than people you kill . . . (*He sits down on the basin rim between his bottles. Consoling himself.*) Have another swig, Marinunzi; don't let them get you down. The fortune-teller saw a boy in her crystal ball; they are easier to bring up than girls; they serve their country, and maybe they can become stars in the sports pages one day . . . You gotta have children to build a great nation. Believing in fortune tellers is a woman's superstition, but at times like these, it helps . . . A great nation . . . When I was single, I paid my dues to the Socialist Party, like everybody else; those four bits, might as well have spent them on drink . . . Now I am for law and order. I am a father, head of a household . . . And as far as order is concerned, we got it now, thanks to a great man who speaks out, and shows the foreigners what's what, and thanks to him, in the next war, we will count. There . . . Where is my bottle? (*He stands up and in so doing spills one of his bottles; he doesn't notice it for he is taken with enthusiasm.*) There's no getting around it; once you drink, you have to drink; you have to roll, to be carried, to lose yourself like with a woman, yet, at the same time, stronger than usual, smarter, braver, more . . . You are the champion, or feel like one . . . You have an empire, like everyone else . . . You inherit Ponte-Porzio . . . Dida croaked . . . Ilario doesn't count anymore . . . Tullia and Maria, you'll be good to them, you'll give them a shack in the back of the garden, what a laugh . . . And it isn't as though there is a shortage of women, if someday, Attilia . . . How nice it is to drink my little wine under my bower, near my gurgling fountain. All the water pipes of Rome can sprout leaks, Oreste Marinunzi couldn't care less. (*He trips, then straightens himself out, then stretches out on the ground.*) Slippery? . . . Damn bottle . . . No, the world is turning . . . The earth is spinning . . . How funny. I am lying down in Ponte-Porzio on the earth that is spinning . . . My place in the sun . . . The bottle is empty, poor bottle . . . I'll damn well have my place in the sun . . . And when I'll wake up . . . And when I'll wake up . . .

(*He snores. It is daylight.*)

END

VITAL STATISTICS

Dida Panicale, born May 2, 1857, Velletri, died August 19, 1938, Ponte-Porzio.

Clément Roux, born August 15, 1860, Hazebrouck (Northern France), died January 12, 1934, Nice.

Giulio Lovisi, born September 2, 1878, Viterbo, died July 11, 1950, Rome.

Paolo Farina, born February 5, 1888, Pietrasanta, died October 17, 1961, Pietrasanta.

Carlo Stevo, born May 19, 1890, Trieste, died April 18, 1933, Lipari Islands.

Alessandro Sarte, born November 9, 1894, Bologna, died March 24, 1944, Ardeatine Caves.

Rosalia di Credo, born November 27, 1895, Gemara (Sicily), died April 20, 1933, Rome.

Father Cicca, born September 2, 1899, Subiaco, died March 24, 1944, Ardeantine Caves.

Giovanna Stevo, born December 1, 1900, Rome, died around 1975, Rome.

Lina Chiari, born May 29, 1901, Florence, died March 30, 1935, Rome.

Marcella Sarte, born June 7, 1904, Cesena, died April 20, 1933, Rome.

Angiola Fides, born December 13, 1904, Gemara (Sicily), died around 1980, Miami.

Maxime Iakovleff, born June 2, 1911, Saint-Petersburg, died May 1, 1945, Auschwitz.

Electra
or
The Fall of The Masks

[1944]

LIST OF CHARACTERS

Electra
Clytemnestra
Aegisthus
Orestes
Pylades
Theodore
Guards

PART I

A whitewashed room. The slits of its door let through the first lights of dawn. Electra is sleeping on the left, on a platform with a mud floor. She has covers over her. A fire is burning in the fireplace flanked by a stone bench. There is a corridor in the foreground leading to the kitchen on the right. Theodore enters cautiously. He is barefooted and is holding a plate of burning coals.

SCENE 1

Theodore, Electra.

THEODORE: Electra! Wake up Electra! It's five o'clock. She is sleeping. She doesn't hear me. Little Electra! Sweet Electra!

ELECTRA: Is that you Theodore? I was just dreaming of a man carrying a bucket of blood.

THEODORE: Don't get so worked up, Electra. It's only the tray of burning coal I bring you every morning so that you won't be cold.

ELECTRA: I'm not cold. I sweat every night.

THEODORE: But you would be cold if I did not get up every time to cover you again after each nightmare.

ELECTRA: (Stroking his head as one strokes a dog.) Yes, you're very kind, you, Theodore.

THEODORE: And I kept a little bowl of oatmeal porridge warm for you on the kitchen stove. It's five o'clock in the morning, Electra. Time for me to go take care of the garden if I want to finish before work at the castle. The North wind blew all night. It's a dry wind that burns the young shoots. And as you know, They wouldn't let me off for a minute to work in my own field, even if the loss of harvest meant that we would go hungry.

ELECTRA: I know that They have no mercy. What day is today, Theodore?

THEODORE: You know what today is, today is Monday.

ELECTRA: Yes, today is Monday; Thursday everything will be decided. You chose this Thursday yourself. And you worry about a small field when we won't be around to see it turn green.

THEODORE: Before one dies, one must live, Electra. And the best thing is perhaps to live exactly as one has always lived. What little courage I have comes from my seedlings and my cuttings. And when I carefully pick a squash from its bed of dry leaves so that it won't rot, I understand better why we are risking death on Thursday.

ELECTRA: Why are you always going on like that? It's not a matter of dying but of killing.

THEODORE: Yes, it's a matter of killing. But he who plays with knives runs the risk of stabbing himself. And it comforts me to think that my sister Ida's children will eat my barley.

ELECTRA: How little you know our enemies! If we fail Thursday your sister Ida and her children will be two feet under the ground, like ourselves.

THEODORE: The plans are laid; we will not fail Thursday. But there are always a few soldiers who don't come back from the battlefield, the unlucky, the clumsy ones. If I turn out to be clumsy this week, Electra, see to it that my sister Ida gets the farm. And I would like to ask you something of more immediate concern. Could you see that the animals are taken care of today? The cow just calved; I can't be everywhere at once. Even if we are avenged Thursday, the animals shouldn't suffer because of it. Aren't you hungry? Aren't you going to eat?

ELECTRA: Throw your porridge to the sow grunting on her bed of straw I forgot to clean. Everything here seems to reproach me; the holes in your clothes, the eyes of your sick cows. Why are you dying for me if what you really care about is this miserable little farm?

THEODORE: It didn't seem so miserable to me in the past. My father was very proud of it after he finished the roof with his own hands.

ELECTRA: Stay on it then and live in peace. You belong to the race of peasants who timidly remove their cap when the master comes by.

THEODORE: No, when the blow has been struck, many poor people like me will be rejoicing in farms all over Argolis. You're not the only one to hate Aegisthus.

ELECTRA: Hating Aegisthus is the only privilege my disasters didn't take from me. I don't intend sharing it with any yokel that comes along.

THEODORE: But me, as soon as I met you, I took my share of your hatred like of a sour apple of which you had the first bite. Your mother's and Aegisthus's crimes were carried out far from me; I was not surprised at rich folk killing each other. I even accepted the wretchedness of the poor. But I saw you digging in the garden, in the rain, bent like an old woman, black and gray like a woman hollowing out the earth for her own grave. Your blistered hands were bleeding; you were wearing a dress a servant would have scorned. That's when I understood injustice.

ELECTRA: Your life is no easier than mine. You deserve better than a Fury in your house.

THEODORE: But I know that your hardness is part of your suffering, as were your chapped hands that night.

ELECTRA: And you came near me in the rain and threw your cloak on my shoulders; it smelled of sheep fat and male sweat. Since Orestes ran away, you were the first human being who spoke to me with kindness. You told me what I had to do when they sent me to work in the fields to get rid of me. And it's to your house I ran, my cheek still red, when Aegisthus slapped me. They said I was a slut chasing the gardener's helper.

THEODORE: God used their slander to allow me to become Electra's guardian and servant. I almost feel like forgiving them.

ELECTRA: And March has gone by five times since then, beginning again the cycle of plowing and planting, but your wife does not bend over new deep furrows with you. The cow calves, the donkey suffers from a wound on her back; you spend the night watching over a sick colt. Your wife does not press the new born lamb against her chest to keep him warm. The bread I knead absentmindedly, almost against my will, comes from the sparse wheat of your little field which you love as my father loved his gardens. I have fed for five years now on the sun of that field, on the wind and dust in your eyes, on the water brought with great pain on your back, or on the donkey's back, on your sweat running on the stones. And you will not harvest the oil of the olive trees your father planted because one day you married a creature not meant for you, the very evening of the day she was thrown out by her mother and her mother's lover. Inspired by a passion for justice, you saw in this wretch a victim of a tyranny even more cowardly than that weighing down the poor. You served me. You are going to avenge me. Perhaps you'll die serving my revenge. But I have never been a good wife to you.

THEODORE: There is one word too many in your last sentence, Electra. You have simply never been a wife to me.

ELECTRA: Don't go back on what was decided, agreed upon that very first night when, leaving the only lamp in the house by my bedside, you went to sleep in a corner of the kitchen. Thus I escaped going from one tyranny to another tyranny, from one egoism to another form of egoism, from a mother to a man. You loved me like a sister.

THEODORE: Perhaps. I can't tell for sure. But you never loved me as you love Orestes.

ELECTRA: That's true. I love Orestes like a child.

THEODORE: And it's because you love Orestes like a child that there is no real child nursing at your breast.

ELECTRA: Are you crazy? By what right could we have a child together?

THEODORE: Sorry, I should not have brought it up. A poor goatkeeper . . . a sharecropper of no consequence . . .

ELECTRA: That's not the point, Theodore. Do soldiers take children along on a dangerous expedition? Does one lie in ambush for an enemy with a child beside him? Leave children to those who are content or resigned. Don't use it as a pretext as they all do. It's because my father mistreated my oldest sister that my mother took a lover, then an ax. What you are thinking about right now is not the lack of a child.

THEODORE: A wife and child. It all goes together, Electra. A wife you sleep with and to whom you tell your dreams in the morning. A child nursing. I can't explain it to you. It's too simple.

ELECTRA: (*Putting her arm around his neck.*) You're the one who is simple, my good Theodore, you're very simple. You're the child. It's right under your nose and you still don't get it. Isn't this murder our child? Wasn't it formed, a shared, unseen secret, heavier and heavier against my heart until you heard it move in me? Aren't the odds that I will die of it covered with blood as though I had given birth? Have you forgotten those long nights spent together in front of the fireplace, side by side, my arm around your neck while your finger outlined in the ashes the lay-out of the castle. Didn't I leave you at dawn my legs just as shaky as those of my mother leaving Aegisthus? And didn't I avert my eyes in the mornings, blushing as though remembering some nocturnal frenzy? Haven't you been happy, Theodore?

THEODORE: Yes, Electra, I have perhaps been as happy as I could.

ELECTRA: Didn't I love you, Theodore?

THEODORE: Yes, Electra. You probably loved me as much as you could.

ELECTRA: Aren't you my friend, Theodore?

(*A knock at the door. Theodore starts up.*)

THEODORE: Quiet. For days now, patrols have been going back and forth on the coastal roads. Someone must have told them of the weapons stockpiled in abandoned quarries.

ELECTRA: You think so? They don't suspect anything.

THEODORE: One never knows. Who's there?

PYLADES' VOICE: A friend.

THEODORE: I'll go. Stay where you are, Electra. Who are you?

PYLADES' VOICE: A friend of Electra.

(*Theodore opens the door and steps back stunned by the arrival of the newcomer. Electra rises.*)

SCENE 2

Theodore, Electra, Pylades.

THEODORE: Already!

ELECTRA: Where is Orestes?

PYLADES: I left him on the beach in case something went wrong. If everything is all right, one of us will go fetch him. If not, the boat was told to wait till noon before lifting anchor.

THEODORE: Ye Gods! It's impossible for us to strike any sooner than planned. Our friends in the castle are not ready.

PYLADES: Did we make a mistake? Electra's last message told us to come Monday at dawn.

ELECTRA: Thursday, Pylades. Didn't I tell them to come Thursday, Theodore?

THEODORE: Could be, Electra. But you forget I don't know how to read.

ELECTRA: Do you suspect me?

THEODORE: Of what could I suspect you, unless it be of wishing to see your brother and his friends two days earlier? But if they notice, from up there, the Argos boat sailing along the coast in broad daylight they'll send search parties out. How will we be able to hide and feed two men for two days?

ELECTRA: Fortunately the path leading to the cistern through the abandoned quarries is perfectly safe.

THEODORE: Yes, no one knows it, not even our friends. Have you ever been there, Pylades?

PYLADES: You took me there early winter during my last visit. I didn't take it this morning, I was afraid of getting lost because there are two ways out.

THEODORE: In case of danger Electra will show you the right way. I'll take that underground path later to lead Orestes to the bottom of the hill. Once there, he'll be able to manage on his own.

ELECTRA: You won't bring him all the way here?

THEODORE: What for? If by some misfortune the alarm is given, it's more important than ever for me to be at the castle at the usual time. I'll try to bring food for you on my way back without arousing suspicion by buying unusual quantities. We have nothing here. You are in the house of poor people.

PYLADES: What commands should Orestes give the boat?

THEODORE: Tell them to come back at the agreed time but in two days.

ELECTRA: No, Theodore. We might need to communicate with the people from Argos. Tell them to send a canoe tonight, at nightfall.

THEODORE: You're right. Goodbye, Pylades. Tonight I'll explain to you both the details of the plan.

(He moves towards the door.)

ELECTRA: Theodore!

THEODORE: (*Turning around.*) What?

ELECTRA: Nothing. Kiss me before you go.

THEODORE: You surprise me, woman. We're not alone.

ELECTRA: Pylades is no stranger. Come. I asked you to kiss me, Theodore.

THEODORE: (*Moved, kisses her.*) All right. I don't really understand. See you tonight Electra.

ELECTRA: Farewell, Theodore.

(*Theodore leaves. Pylades sits down on the bench in front of the hearth.*)

SCENE 3

Electra, Pylades.

PYLADES: Who's mistaken here, or who's being betrayed, Electra?

ELECTRA: In any case, not you.

PYLADES: You really asked us to come today?

ELECTRA: Yes, today.

PYLADES: For three years now Theodore has been the messenger going between Argos and you. He must have crossed the gulf and mountain of Argos at least twenty times through storms and squalls. He's the one who had the good sense to prevent Orestes from joining you last year when you were asking for your brother. He's the one who brought you, half carried you, to Argolis when you absolutely had to see him after that last attack of fever. It's thanks to him that we could keep contact with our friends in town who will make our return easier. It seems to me that you could trust him as much as you trust me and even more.

ELECTRA: It's precisely because I respect Theodore's integrity that I don't reveal my plans to him.

PYLADES: You surprise me. After all, it's not a matter of sticking up a cashier and dividing the loot among us.

ELECTRA: Theodore has been thinking about this act of justice now for three years, and he has not come up with anything better than scaling up the castle wall in the middle of the night with the help of a groggy caretaker and two or three guards. And in this plan, I am to play no part whatsoever. Yet, you can't both be killed without me.

PYLADES: What you mean is that we can't kill them without you. Theodore is wrong to keep the she-wolf from joining in the kill.

ELECTRA: Theodore still has illusions about the tender heartedness of women. And those are not his only prejudices.

PYLADES: Which others?

ELECTRA: His imagination does not go further than simple murder; it never carries him as far as the ambush.

PYLADES: And it's this ambush that you've plotted to take place in his absence?

ELECTRA: Yes, here, this afternoon. In this room. She is coming to be reconciled with me after five years of absence; she'll rub her make-up against my cheeks, commiserate with me about this sordid marriage she forced me into. She'll feel sorry for me because of this miserable hovel she makes me live in, she'll notice with joy that I am more faded at twenty-five than she at forty-seven. She'll come alone. She's not afraid. She might even bring me some rum and jam in a basket. Now that she is getting older, she likes to play the lady of the castle among the poor. I saw her from afar two or three times walking on the road to Nauplia with a pink parasol above her head. She had no one with her, not even a servant. And the children of the village cling to her skirts as Orestes and I used to do when we were small.

PYLADES: They say she does good deeds. She is probably popular.

ELECTRA: Women like her always succeed with men and children of the poor.

PYLADES: You're wrong, Electra; there are clumsy prostitutes.

ELECTRA: And since they have taken upon themselves to help me by repairing my roof, the rack of the donkey, the latrines in the courtyard, Aegisthus will come to fetch her in person, the practical man, to examine everything with her. You understand? One after the other.

PYLADES: He's never without an escort.

ELECTRA: He'll leave his escort behind, with his carriage, at the bottom of the hill. He won't want to look ridiculous in the eyes of his wife and step-daughter. I'm telling you they don't distrust me. They think my spirit is broken. Me, broken, imagine! And even if he put two sleepy guards by the porch in the garden, there will always be a way to strike him on the cellar stairs and to escape by the quarries before the alarm is given. We'll just have to act fast, that's all.

PYLADES: Is it to act fast that you gave the boat the order to come back this very evening?

ELECTRA: Yes, if all goes well, we'll be on the other side of the gulf before dawn tomorrow.

PYLADES: Your plan is good but I see one risk. If the second part of the project fails, if the man doesn't come, the death of that fat sloppy woman solves nothing, and we will be disgraced.

ELECTRA: I don't get it.

PYLADES: I thought as much. Our own crimes and vices are always nameless to us; it's a rather unpleasant experience to find out what the public calls them. What you and Orestes are going to commit here is called matricide.

ELECTRA: I call it an act of justice.

PYLADES: What did you do to prepare this act of justice? Did you make up with them? Did you promise wine and honey?

ELECTRA: Simpler than that. I wrote to them that I was pregnant.

PYLADES: Are you pregnant?

ELECTRA: Look at me from profile. Do I look as if I were expecting?

PYLADES: No, thin as a rail, or a blade. Ah, I'm also beginning to be amused by the approach of the decisive moment. Give me your hands, sister of Orestes.

ELECTRA: (*Giving him her hands.*) What for? Do you want to read my future? Is my life line short?

PYLADES: Longer than the line of your heart, wife of Theodore. Do you realize that Theodore is your scapegoat? He'll come home here tonight, not suspecting a thing, at the precise moment all the policemen of Mycenes will be on the lookout. Our friends will be the first to abandon him, only too happy to sacrifice an insignificant victim to popular emotion. The odds are you will be the widow of a martyr by tomorrow.

ELECTRA: Theodore runs risks just like us all.

PYLADES: And the kiss you gave him in front of me was that a compensation?

ELECTRA: Let go of my wrists. What gives you the right to butt into my life?

PYLADES: The right that every convict has to know his chain gang companion. I'm sure that last kiss was also the first.

ELECTRA: I only lie to my mother, Pylades, and only to punish her for having lied so much herself. The kiss you're speaking of was the first kiss.

PYLADES: Perfect! You never struck me as the kind of woman able to make love to a farmer, in a barn.

ELECTRA: And this is the man I entrusted Orestes to!

PYLADES: Maybe you were wrong entrusting Orestes to me, my dear. I have no father to avenge. Frankly, if it were only a matter of reclaiming my possessions confiscated by Aegisthus, I'd rather forget the whole story, black and dry like curdled blood. I'd go try my luck in Sidon or Carthage. Do you know why I let myself be dragged along in this unsavory enterprise?

ELECTRA: You are Orestes' friend.

PYLADES: That's right; I am Orestes' friend. Did it ever cross your mind that the brother could lead to the sister?

ELECTRA: What you're insinuating would make me laugh were I capable of laughing on the day that will decide of Orestes' life and of their death. Nothing ever proved to me that you would have given me another role in your narrow friendship than that of a servant which is the one that suits older sisters. You have hardly seen me more than two or three times since the day I entrusted Orestes to you, an Orestes sick from the escape, from the rough traveling, from the memory of the recent murder and from the horrible hypocritical tenderness that bloodied twosome bestowed on him. You know how weak he is, how easily manipulated, how fragile. When I saw that the beatings were for me and the caresses for him, I understood that he had to be saved at all cost. Just think: a twelve-year-old child and these wretches tried to make him an accomplice of their crime, tried to make him part of their adultery. The man showered him with gifts and gave him holidays, and the woman, sniffling by his bed, kissed him with her mouth still warm from Aegisthus. That's when I thought of you; you were the only family I knew safely settled outside of Mycenes. I can still see our nocturnal arrival in your house in Argos, your father half rising from his couch, a sick man, your big clumsy boyish hands lifting up Orestes' head, finding the right gesture to cover him with a jacket, to press a glass of water to his lips. And these words of friendship no girls can make up. And me, of whom you speak today as if I were somebody, me on the threshold, my hand in the hand of the old servant who had led our expedition, me, hardly noticed, ready to go back to my hell.

PYLADES: Who made you? My father was ready to treat you like a daughter.

ELECTRA: Let's say that my presence and Orestes' absence was the best torture I could cook up for them, up there.

PYLADES: Or more simply, you wanted to suffer.

ELECTRA: If that's the case, I had my fill; I suffered. I suffered from the beatings, the cold food, the work I had to do with the servants. I suffered being alone, separated, suffered that a thirteen-year-old boy took so long to grow up. I suffered at the thought that he and I could die, stupidly, before having paid them back, wound for wound, sneer for sneer, spit for spit. The absence of that boy was both my masterpiece and my agony; he was safe and I was alone to weep by myself. It wasn't me anymore but you who comforted him in his despair, who allayed his doubts, who helped him, hour after hour, to prepare his future. He traded an older sister for an older brother. Ah, you'll never know with what mixture of gratitude and jealousy I thought of you.

PYLADES: Forget your gratitude and don't complicate everything with your jealousy. You have been stronger than your brother, tougher than myself. If Orestes and I came to your house this morning to kill, and if those two come later to die, it's because you have been standing still in one place, slowly secreting the cobweb threads of fate. You never left Argos. Your secret messengers maintained your presence there like muted stifled cries coming out of an oppressed homeland. We learned of the execution of the old servant who had lead you to us; we knew you were being beaten, starved, forced by your wretchedness into a grotesque marriage. Orestes wept about it all night long in his bed, less out of love for you than pity and horror for his fallen family. He suffered from your misfortunes as if he had been a woman in your place. The longer I lived at his side, the more I took responsibilities for him, responsibilities that aged me, an only son, turned into the oldest brother. The more I lived mingled to his tears, his sudden laughter, his crazy despair, his tender egoism typical of protected victims, the more I felt that this weak mouth, this fragile body evoked another more enduring body, a harder mouth. I saw you together again; I compared the two faces—yours was more virile; I saw you breathe your hatred into him as one breathes a strident music into a reed. I saw you put plans for the future into his hands, over and over again, as one keeps picking up a toy and handing it back to an indolent child who keeps on dropping it.

ELECTRA: Do you think you're winning me by insulting my brother? And I thought you were his friend!

PYLADES: Didn't I love your brother? Didn't I waste my patrimony for him? Wasn't I glad my father died, which is another way of committing patricide, because his death allowed me to give Orestes my whole fortune? Haven't I traded the role of a banker's son for that of an outlaw, because of him? Have I done anything else these last ten years except to think of Orestes? Some people are loved for their weakness, Electra, others for their strength; I'm here for Orestes but because of Electra.

ELECTRA: I don't care why you are here as long as you don't hesitate, as long as you strike just slowly enough for them to see themselves dying, but quick enough for them not being able to call for help. Do you realize that probably at this very moment she is getting up or she is still talking to him from her bed while he is bending over his little mirror to shave? Now she is choosing her dress, the very dress she'll come to dazzle me in later. Neither one of them suspects that they are getting dressed for the last time.

PYLADES: And do you understand that if our severed heads are not displayed tonight on the Lioness' Gate, we will have to go on for some twenty, thirty years after this butcher's task? What are you going to do with these twenty years, young Electra? Will you live as an old maid cherishing the memory of an outdated murder? Will you live haunted by thirty minutes of crime as others are by a lovers' stroll in the garden? The fat, bloated woman getting up right now at least has had money, power and ten years of sleeping with Aegisthus. Are you going to be satisfied forever with the minor role of the sister, and me, the doubtful one of the friend? Have you ever thought that once the little upcoming formality has been accomplished, we take legal possession of caves full of gold and barricaded with iron, of ships swollen with Egyptian wheat, Cyprus spices, that is to say, the powers that make the world go round. Two ghosts are going to settle accounts with other ghosts tonight, and suddenly your nightmarish life becomes brutally, innocently real. You only get rid of the dead if you can replace them. Haven't you ever felt like taking your morning bath in that infamous bathtub, scoured so clean that no telltale blood stains remain? Wouldn't you like to lie tonight on royal tiger skins, fully dressed, like a young soldier sleeping amid the loot?

ELECTRA: Be quiet. Leave me the illusion that the battle is pure.

PYLADES: You make too much of purity, cold Electra. Two bodies exposed to the same dangers can roll on the same bed with as much innocence as in the same grave.

ELECTRA: Don't remind me that I have just sent the only man who had the right to own me to his death with the worst of kisses as last sacrament.

PYLADES: Nonsense! You advanced his death by two days so as to avoid a couple of nights disturbed by the demands of a dying man. Because in times like these, even the weak can become violent, and the stupid, persuasive. Are you sure that you only thought of your brother's and my security, prudent Electra?

ELECTRA: No! No! Theodore is loyal, he is pure; he loves me as a dog or as a bridegroom; he asks God only for my happiness. Besides, remember that you see before you a disgraced, ugly girl. My mother said I was swarthy; Aegisthus made fun of my nose, of my eyes.

PYLADES: Do I look like the kind of a man who would risk his life for a pretty face? The mirrors of the palace will teach you the exact degree of your ugliness tomorrow, modest Electra.

ELECTRA: To think that we're the pure ones, the just, those the poets will pity, those who hold celestial vengeance in their hands! I almost envy them, those two miserable creatures we shall kill. And indeed, what am I going to do but to remove them from this confusion, this infamy, and allow them to become as pure in death as was the corpse of my father, hands folded, on the edge of his grave?

PYLADES: Don't delude yourself about the purity of the dead; they rot very quickly, naive Electra. And those receiving or giving the last stroke hardly have enough time to savor it. Aegisthus' little grimace will disappoint you later.

ELECTRA: I won't be disappointed. I'm doing it for Orestes.

PYLADES: Don't have too many illusions about Orestes, older sister. I love him more than you do since I know his weaknesses better. Love of Orestes justifies for us all crimes, all marriages. He will always need your lap to rest his head on, my shoulder to lean on. I can't picture a single morning of our life where we won't have to take care of Orestes. Tomorrow he will be our excuse in the eyes of the people the way he had been your pretext these last ten years. Your brother is a sort of first child between us.

ELECTRA: Enough! I've already heard words to that effect whispered around Orestes' cradle. It's such pretexts that Aegisthus must have used with my mother.

PYLADES: Don't worry, little Electra, we'll get rid of your mother for you. You won't have to spend your life looking at yourself in the deforming mirror of this woman grown flabby with age. You'll be able to take a lover without remembering that your mother lived in sin. And don't compare me to Aegisthus, or Agamemnon with Theodore. We'll get rid of Aegisthus for you. We'll just allow him five deadly seconds to repent for having made fun of your nose and eyes. You'll be able to trample his hands, to pull his gray hair.

ELECTRA: (Ecstatic, letting herself go.) You won't miss, will you! Oh, how good vengeance will be! How good to be able to admit that one hungers for vengeance and not only justice! I couldn't, I couldn't with Theodore.

PYLADES: (*Sitting down next to her, touching her hair.*) And your hands are clenched like those of an athlete about to jump, your blood is burning in your forehead and under your hair. I saw boys shake with excitement, like you now, at the prospect of a boxing match. But you have yet to learn how to economize your strength before the crime. Look how you're trembling.

ELECTRA: Sh . . . I hear Orestes' footsteps on the stairs leading from the cistern. He stumbles on the same step I stumble on every morning. Oh! Blessed be the naked feet of the Avenger! Leave me, Pylades. I must go, I must show him.

PYLADES: Your brother arrives and you draw back from me like an accomplice. There is a secret between us.

ELECTRA: Three friends can share six secrets, two by two, Pylades.

(*Orestes appears on the threshold of the door. He's covered with dust and he's very pale.*)

SCENE 4

Electra, Pylades, Orestes.

ORESTES: Don't come near me, Electra. I'm covered with the dust of your cellar's staircase. How awful, this winding underground path! Right at the spot Theodore left me, where the road sinks between two sides of the mountain, I turned around to look behind me at the sea and the hills of the Gulf of Argos. It's probably the last time I will look at the sea with innocent eyes.

PYLADES: Spare us your eloquence. So, when you leave here, you will look at the sea with eyes of a criminal for the first time.

ORESTES: (*Sitting down before the hearth.*) And this house! Pylades had told me that you lived on the most deserted, exposed side of the mountain, but one can never really imagine anything. I didn't picture these cracked walls, this chipped plate in the ashes, this sow in the kitchen courtyard. And to think that I lived in Argos in a palace surrounded by gardens! Pylades took me to the Olympian races, to the Delphi festivals. I ate at the house of the princes of Athens. And you, my older sister, you tried to keep warm with this miserable little ember fire.

ELECTRA: Don't feel too sorry for me, Orestes. I didn't see this house. I wasn't conscious of the cold in winters, or the heat in summers. I had my own seasons, my own dark sun, my poisoned fruit ripening on secret vines. This squalid room wasn't any dirtier than our unavenged lives. I ended up loving it, taking it for the snake pit, for the sheath of Electra's knife. I decorated these walls with huge red frescoes.

PYLADES: Not so frantic, Electra, you're scaring the child.

ORESTES: But how did you manage to live here, to eat here, to lean over a mirror to braid your hair? Now I understand why you are as dark as a peasant woman, why your sweet voice is hoarse, like a raspy fruit of fireless winters. And this bitterness that had saddened me during your visits to Argos—that comes only from suffering. Your house, my poor sister, smells of wild beasts and of death, like a trap and a tomb.

PYLADES: We didn't know you had the gift of clairvoyance, Orestes. The future, like the past, must have its ghosts, especially when the future is only a few hours away. Electra's house is a trap; it is going to be a tomb.

ORESTES: (Rising.) Ah! Sister more than sister. Friend almost brother. Have we been betrayed? Do we have to die?

PYLADES: Explain, Electra. Don't let him strike up an elegy for himself.

ELECTRA: Why must every act always be more disgraceful than hoped for, be smaller than expected? He dreamed of an ambush outdoors under the stars, in an unblemished night. Tell him, if you can, that the enemy can be killed more conveniently between four walls.

PYLADES: Aegisthus and your mother are coming this very day. The event, the act of justice as Electra calls it, will take place in this room. Electra will welcome them on the threshold. We'll hide behind this door.

ORESTES: Here in this room, behind this door?

ELECTRA: Yes, my Orestes. For once they won't be surrounded by the police and the gold of Mycenes. They won't appear as the great and rich people they seemed to us when we were poor little children. And therein lies their real death, in that plunge from the heights of their prestige; in this humility of casual strollers entering, as if by chance, the inn where justice awaits them. We won't miss. They'll die like anybody else.

PYLADES: Will you tell him what pretext you used to obtain this little family visit, Electra?

ELECTRA: No, Pylades. My lie is of no interest to Orestes.

ORESTES: Here, in this room, behind this door. I'll never be able to do it . . .

PYLADES: Do you think it's easier to strangle guards?

ORESTES: I'll never be able to. I'll never be able to wait behind that door. I remember having played those games of hide-and-seek. I was hiding in the dark, behind a door, my mother was looking for me. She was looking for her son in the dark.

PYLADES: Childhood memories are impressive only in books, Orestes. Seeing that we have been talking about it for so long, you should have gotten used to the idea of killing your mother.

ORESTES: I got used to the idea of killing a woman lying on the royal bed with my father's murderer, with the usurper stealing our inheritance, with the tyrant tormenting our friends. I had gotten used to doing battle by sword, at night, when you don't know who you're killing. I surely can't kill her if I see her so close. She'll have the same gestures she used to have. Maybe she'll even have around her neck the same crystal trinket I liked putting in my mouth. I surely can't kill her if I remember that I am her child.

ELECTRA: You won't recognize her. She has gotten horribly fat.

PYLADES: You're not going to lecture us on blood ties like some melodramatic hero? And in a quivering voice, you'll remind us later that she carried you in her belly for nine months.

ORESTES: It's not a question of her belly. It's not a question of her heart. And if my mother carried me nine months, I don't remember. Nor do I remember the time she nursed me before turning me over to a wet nurse because it was easier. But I do remember that she taught me to wash myself, and helped me to learn how to read. You can't expect me to be able to kill the woman who showed me how to use a knife and a spoon.

PYLADES: That won't be necessary. You won't have to kill her. We'll only need a hand with Aegisthus.

ELECTRA: No, Pylades, it will be necessary. There are fools all over the world. Do you think that I want to undertake what they call a crime all by myself? I will have toiled five years to give Orestes his title back, his fortune—to wash him clean of any suspicion that he, the only son, could have made common cause with the murderers of his father. And now the boy would simply stand by while I finish the dirty work all alone? And tomorrow, he would be able to lift towards the sky hands more like young girl's than mine are, hands still pure? No, what is going to occur here is a sort of Mass in which everyone must participate. It really is a matter of blood ties.

PYLADES: And besides, she's not your mother anymore, she's Aegisthus' wife. For ten years now, the only children that would have mattered were those she fortunately did not bring into the world.

ELECTRA: (Crossing herself.) In the name of the father. In the name of the son. Yes, God punished their adultery by making them sterile.

ORESTES: She'll come here, flushed, out of breath from having climbed up in the wind. I could no more kill her than I could kill my nurse were she accused of misconduct with the cook.

PYLADES: Remember that if our plan fails today we can look forward to returning humbly to our friends in Argos or Athens. Pity for the losers, and subsidies for the banished don't last forever. Are you really bent on playing forever the role of a parasite who has known better times?

ORESTES: You understand, Electra, it's not a question of filial love. Even before her crime, I did not love my mother. Does a child love? What I loved was to sit on her big lap, to seek shelter, in her skirts, from the sea wind blowing on the Eastern terrace. I loved the warm spot left in her bed right after she got up, and the noise her amber bracelet made on her left arm when it hit against her gold one. And I hated her breath on my porridge, her kisses against my ear, and that horrible smell of perfume and soap on her hands after she had just washed them. It's this collection of pleasures and aversions that I remember, and not my mother.

ELECTRA: And is your compassionate heart also moved by Aegisthus? The two of you won't be too many to kill that man.

ORESTES: I will kill Aegisthus as one fires a butler caught stealing, a coachman who doesn't know his trade. I feel nothing for Aegisthus, not even hatred. I'll get rid of him as one throws a stone into the waters, careful only not to get splashed. Does Aegisthus really exist? Any stable groom could be Aegisthus to a forty-year-old matron.

PYLADES: He will eliminate you unless you eliminate him. I call that existing.

ELECTRA: Does he exist? My cheek still bears the mark of Aegisthus' slap, and my wrist his fingerprints and the mark where he wrung my arm one day, trying to make me confess where I had hidden you. And our father is rotting in his tomb, his forehead gashed by Aegisthus. I never saw a woodcutter fell an oak, I never heard that awful deafening noise announcing the death of a tree without thinking of the cracking sound the ax made on the nape of that giant who fell, caught in the folds of his bathrobe, blinded by the rising steam.

ORESTES: Enough! I have enough nightmares to remember all that. But even those nightmares are made up of memories told, of memories that were not my own. For my part, I remember Aegisthus as a clumsy stranger, a little shy, speaking to me in a ridiculous grown-up voice, as one speaks to the children of the hostess who has invited you for dinner. A visitor who stuck up for me when my mother would scold me. A great friend who sent me to the Nauplia fair to ride on the carousel.

ELECTRA: And do you know why you were sent to that village fair? His servant had orders to bring you back only at twilight, the deed accomplished, when they would have had time to wash the bathroom pavement and to calm down the hysterical maids. I can still see you coming home, your hands full of gingerbreads and penny toys, frightened, worried by the whispers and the silence, as soon as you stepped through the door—you, the innocent one, like a child who misbehaved. And she who will come later, told you to speak softly because your father was very sick; she didn't admit right away that your father was dead.

ORESTES: She bent down to kiss me. I still remember her cheek, so warm and trembling. I touched it; I asked her if she was ill. He was looking the other way, embarrassed as though ashamed.

ELECTRA: Well, they weren't ashamed in front of me; they didn't use pious lies. I saw everything. No, I didn't see, I heard. I heard my father dying. The bathroom door had been left ajar to clear the steam a little. I heard the sound of the sword-belt, and the shoes dropping, one by one, on the floor; and the pleased laughter of the soldier come back home, amazed to find all his brushes in place, his shaving kit intact. I saw a woman's arm coming through the opening of the door to take the towel I was offering, me, the little girl delighted to be useful. And the false note of cheerfulness in that voice exclaiming "There's something wrong with the heat. Come look, Aegisthus." And that awful struggle on the wet pavement, and the way she came out. And the way she held back the door, looking to make sure no one was coming in the corridor, torn between the wish to go back inside to help her lover and the fear of catching a blow that would disfigure her. And me, I was there, too petrified to scream but opening my mouth wide, as if I were listening with my throat, trying to separate one sound from the other, both of them so close, the sound of water leaving the bathtub and the rattle of a father dying. She was staring at me—she didn't stop staring at me. I'm sure she was glad I was there. I was there so often. I saw her let Aegisthus put his arms around her waist on the garden bench, I saw her leaving Aegisthus' room in the morning, finishing Aegisthus' glass of wine on the side-board. To learn everything, I had put my ear to the wall of her room; I heard her gurgle with pleasure in Aegisthus' arms. And now she was happy to force me to hear that rattle, to see the blood seeping under the door; she was getting even with me as much as with Agamemnon.

ORESTES: And you took me by the hand and led me to the Armory where they had placed him; in the other hand you had a night-lamp. He was so terribly big and so awfully pale. As you held me against you, both of them came running, and they stayed by my bedside the whole night because I was sobbing so loud.

ELECTRA: They fixed it so that the blows could not be seen. He seemed at peace, as though removed from harm. Thoughtful as a church statue. Calm as a God.

ORESTES: I saw him only when he was dead. I was too young to remember his brief visits between two battles, and I hardly caught a glimpse of him between the flags unfurling the morning of the crime. But I remember the portraits pinned on farm walls, passed from hand to hand on victory days.

ELECTRA: They killed him still young, ready for other battles, ripe for other victories that would have justified the first ones. Without him the world drags from war to war, grotesque as a blind man who lost his guide. Because a wicked woman took a lover, Greece lost its only chance for peace.

ORESTES: I don't give a damn about Greece. I don't give a damn about the world. Let each orphan cope with a loss or an absence. But what did they do to us, his children.

ELECTRA: They married the daughter to shame, the son to exile. They made the daughter into a wild beast growling in her lair.

ORESTES: They made a tramp out of Orestes, a vagabond roaming foreign lands, begging for tears and smiles, sullied by compromises—a son looking for a fragment of the broken father in each protector. They turned all my loves into attempts to escape, all friends into accomplices. They forced me to be like them. I wanted to be like the other one, the dead man, the one who only fought in broad daylight, who suspected nothing, who, not having suffered, did not need to be avenged, and who died like a lion on the day of his first encounter with a human trap. They made every woman into a mask of betrayal and horror for me so that they squashed in me his chance of having heirs. They will turn us into murderers. They force us to wait for them behind a door, ax in hand, as they waited for my father.

ELECTRA: They killed God, the only God children understand, the God in whose image they imagine God.

ORESTES: Since I hardly knew him, for me he was more than a man. Sitting in the light of the hearth, at night, Aegisthus with his tired hands was my image of a man. That's why I can't hate this Aegisthus I want to obliterate. That's why I'm not crying over my father. Does one really cry for a father? Maybe I would have hated my father had he lived. I cried because Aegisthus had killed my God, and I was scared—the God the maids told me to fear and to imitate, the distant Almighty who punished me when I misbehaved.

ELECTRA: They destroyed happiness. They annihilated innocence. Isn't that enough for us to kill them in our turn, my poor brother?

ORESTES: It's enough to wish for their death. And it's enough to wish to die, to hide underground, like Him, to flee from a world where order does not rule.

ELECTRA: Our father who art in his tomb,

ORESTES: Thy will be done,

ELECTRA: Our vengeance come,

ORESTES: And forgive us our sins,

ELECTRA: Since we do not forgive those who have sinned against us.

PART II

The same stage set. It's the afternoon of the same day. The door in the back is open showing the arid countryside and the citadel of Mycenes on the horizon. Lying down, carefully wrapped up in blankets, Electra unbraids her hair.

SCENE 1

Electra, then Clytemnestra.

ELECTRA: In this country, it is the custom for women in labor to unbraid their hair before giving birth. They want no knot on them. Nothing to interrupt or to stop the future. There . . . Under all these blankets pulled up to my chin, she won't be able to tell that my chest is flat and my belly unswollen. Nor will she notice the knife against my thigh. The door is open. All she has left to do now is to come in as though she were home. She'll come up to my bed, she'll sit on this stool and I'll turn my head towards her, slowly as though I were in pain. Perhaps she'll take my hand; she'll be moved by my plight. They say two women are easily tender with each other when they're alone. In this corridor, Orestes and his friend, my brother and my friend, are waiting like midwives to bring justice into the world. Orestes drank to give himself courage—he won't waver: he will carry out his task to the end. Ah, mother darling, is something within you, wiser than yourself, shuddering and guessing what's going to happen, and despairing because your body and your mind ignore it? Do your realize that you have eaten your last breakfast, slept with Aegisthus for the last time? Perhaps you are blaming your stomach or your heart for your palpitations? And you're worried about your change of life. Don't be afraid, Mother, don't be so afraid that you won't come. Come, Mother, come see your daughter. If you didn't come, I think I would die of disappointment and shame. Oh, the fear and joy of waiting for Orestes were not as sweet and dreadful as this particular waiting. What! What's that? I hear the sound of high heels on the stones . . . a rustle of silk against the bushes. Thank God, thank God, thank God! What? What did you say? I'm speaking too loud? I'm allowed to speak out loud to myself. I'm allowed to speak out loud to my child.

CLYTEMNESTRA: (*Standing in the threshold, hesitates to come in.*) Daughter! Daughter Electra.

ELECTRA: Mother. You can't see. You are afraid. It doesn't matter. You'll get used to the dark. You've come to see your daughter? How I have waited for you mother, every single day for five years I waited for you.

CLYTEMNESTRA: My poor Electra!

ELECTRA: Do you feel sorry for me? Do you feel sorry for your daughter? You feel sorry for my living in this smoke-filled hut, for giving birth on this straw mattress under these rags? You're ashamed of me, Mother, aren't you? Close the door. Come sit here on this stool. Let me touch your silk dress. It's been such a long time since I've touched silk, real silk that screams when it is torn.

CLYTEMNESTRA: Are you near your term? Are you afraid?

ELECTRA: The closer I get to my term, the less I'm afraid.

CLYTEMNESTRA: Does he treat you well? Does he make you happy? In bed, gardener's helper can equal a prince.

ELECTRA: In those things, you're the expert, mother, not I.

CLYTEMNESTRA: Sharp tongue. I see my Electra hasn't changed. If you're on a straw mattress you have only your pride to blame.

ELECTRA: The poverty you're seeing is your handiwork. Your Aegisthus made me this gardener's wife you see.

CLYTEMNESTRA: Can I blame Aegisthus to want to rid us of a snake? He never forgave you Orestes' flight.

ELECTRA: Yes, his rights seemed less secure when he could no longer pass himself off as the heir's tutor.

CLYTEMNESTRA: Nothing gave you the right to abduct my child.

ELECTRA: That's the first time you have shown a mother's heart.

CLYTEMNESTRA: I've not reached forty without judging myself, without knowing that I could have done better, that perhaps one single gesture would have changed it all. If I had hugged you more, if I had taught you to trust your mother, you would not have grown up into this she-wolf. But I loved Orestes passionately, stupidly, clumsily and madly. When he was a baby his crying was a music that prevented me from smelling his swaddling clothes. You're not a mother yet, my daughter; perhaps you'll understand when you'll hold in your arms, not your first, but your last born.

ELECTRA: Your love for Orestes did not prevent you from preferring your lover and your vengeance to him.

CLYTEMNESTRA: Are you aware of the weight that cradle had on my life? It's Orestes' little hands that I saw that evening while I was sharpening the ax against the grindstone in the garden.

ELECTRA: Indeed. The existence of a male heir guaranteed you the right of succession and allowed you to be widowed without worrying.

CLYTEMNESTRA: You insist on seeing your father's death as some sort of feast Aegisthus and I gave ourselves. You'll never know the hurts that gave birth to hatred or the sufferings that brought forth revenge. Our crime was a bloody amputation, and your stepfather and I were two patients who had to choose between death and surgery.

ELECTRA: And where did that gangrene come from? I know that any friend who betrays his friend begins a murder, and that any woman who lets herself be seduced starts an abortion or an infanticide. You killed my father during your very first tryst with Aegisthus.

CLYTEMNESTRA: What you say would be true if one were really clear-sighted at those moments when the heart, drowning in pleasure, trembles like a water lily on a pond ruffled by a breeze—and the present is stronger than the future because it is sweeter than the past. Women weep with their eyes open my daughter but they make love with their eyes closed.

ELECTRA: Tell me, mother. Did he love you that much? Were you that crazy about him?

CLYTEMNESTRA: He was everything life gave as compensation. He was the explanation for it all: that one could love love, want a child, risk all one has in order to live or die together.

ELECTRA: And did that great love last? Is it still that lamp that goes on, unfailingly, every night for you? Do you still lie down every night in it, still rise from it every morning?

CLYTEMNESTRA: Nothing lasts without change. This love is all life left me after your machinations took Orestes from me. He's still the best thing in the world that I have.

ELECTRA: And you're faithful to him. No other man in your life these last five years?

CLYTEMNESTRA: One can't keep anything from you, my daughter. Two or three times perhaps. Guests, friends of Aegisthus. One wants to be reassured that one is still beautiful, that Aegisthus still has reasons for loving.

ELECTRA: Mother! So, even a great love is not enough.

CLYTEMNESTRA: A great love contains everything even the crimes against itself. It's like a sea in which you can drown or piss, but neither corpses or urine change the color of the water.

ELECTRA: So it was pure luck that no other Aegisthus took over your sheets or the keys to the safe? Aegisthus in his turn could come in contact with the sharp side of an ax and the pavement of the bathroom?

CLYTEMNESTRA: You need love and hate to do what I did, and of the two, hate is perhaps the most needed ingredient. You don't hate like that twice in one lifetime.

ELECTRA: You had no right to make us the children of such hate.

CLYTEMNESTRA: I didn't always hate him. Your father wasn't always this brute whose unexpected returns scared the children and the servants.

ELECTRA: And what were you but an unfaithful servant? We, his children, were not scared.

CLYTEMNESTRA: No, you flourished in this quarrelsome atmosphere, and Orestes, at the kite flying and marble playing age, did not suspect danger.

ELECTRA: And what dangers threatened Orestes when he was with his father?

CLYTEMNESTRA: You can expect the worst from a man brutalized by ten years of war, of colonial occupation, of depredation, burned by fevers, rotting from diseases that are nameless here.

ELECTRA: You're blaming the chief for the misfortunes of his calling. His duties detained him in Asia.

CLYTEMNESTRA: Speak to the people about his honorable duties! We knew that his dreams of ambition and personal gain were the only reasons for prolonging a useless war by ten years. Everyone here knew that he profited as much from every defeat as from a victory.

ELECTRA: You're lying. I was old enough to see tears in his eyes when he spoke of dead soldiers.

CLYTEMNESTRA: But he was much more interested in the live mistresses he picked up in Asian brothels.

ELECTRA: And you yourself were so pure, weren't you? Your marital fidelity gave you the right to judge him? Your own assignations with Aegisthus were really clean, weren't they, these little trysts in the courtyard sentry box that's like a wooden coffin for a soldier or for a twosome standing up. Your back blocked the entry. All I saw of him were two clutching hands; your head hung back, assailed, at times, by a stubborn fly.

CLYTEMNESTRA: That scream in the wind, that was you? You were spying on your mother!

ELECTRA: And were the other rendez-vous any cleaner, those meetings in the linen room when the maids had gone back to their garrets to meet their own lovers? I was looking for my sick little cat everywhere. I can still see that big empty room, soiled linen in a corner, a body white in the moonlight, a man frightened, propping himself up on his right elbow.

CLYTEMNESTRA: So, that little mouse that startled us, that was you? And who forced you to play the sniffing animal, nose to the ground? Your loyalty towards your father or the curiosity of an adolescent girl?

ELECTRA: I needed no pretexts or excuses. Can you imagine the unhappiness of a child afraid to open the door to the cellar, or to walk into the garden pavilion lest she should stumble on her mother entwined with a man?

CLYTEMNESTRA: And you were completely absorbed in your research weren't you? And you would hide, all excited, in my closet or under my bed. And when you heard Aegisthus' footsteps in the corridor your body shook more than mine, the lover. And you stretched your head, your chest half sticking out of your hiding place, risking the shame of being discovered for a better look at Aegisthus' arms entering the sleeves of the shirt I had embroidered for him. But afterwards you did not fall asleep as we did; you did not go, like us, from an evening of passion to a happy night. How many times did you regret that your hands were too small to strangle us? And how many times did you wake up all flustered from your dreams of Aegisthus? How many times did you think of Aegisthus while you were in the arms of your gardener? How right I was to mistrust your comings and goings in the corridor in the morning, and your short little girl skirts that showed your skinny legs, and your eyes stubbornly lowered but seeking out Aegisthus. How you envied me my lover! And how, weeping for your father's death, you managed to crumble on the couch, showing with each sob a bit more naked shoulder.

ELECTRA: Bitch, cow, pig! Shut up. Will she shut up? Shut up, I said. Ah, let me get my hands around her fat neck, let me shake those fat cheeks to keep her from speaking.

CLYTEMNESTRA: But I am speaking, I'm screaming, and what I say I will repeat in a minute for Aegisthus. And your father was a disgusting slob, an idiot, a dirty brute dirtier right after his bath than my naked lover after an hour of love. And you, with your hysterical tears and your dirty little girl vices! What a pair you made, the two of you. We were cleansed by adultery as by a baptism. And I've been happy, happier than you will ever be on top of your dung-hill with your village rooster. And your father got what he deserved, the old torturer, the old rotting traitor. And Orestes' father . . .

ELECTRA: Oh shut up. I make her shut up with my hands. I shove the words back in her throat. Let them burst like bubbles. They smell. She's looking at me. Her face is bright red. Have her shut up. Friend! Friend! Hold her hands. Flabby all over, warm, her double chin quivering.

SCENE 2

Electra, Pylades.

PYLADES: (*Entering the room.*) Let me see, Electra. You managed quite well on your own. Now your mother no longer loves Aegisthus, nor suffers from varicose veins, nor prefers mint sauce to thyme sauce, nor pale blue to purple. What's the matter with you? Are you fainting?

ELECTRA: Did you hear? Did you hear what my mother was saying to me?

PYLADES: Forget it. The living speak with voices and the voice is still what disappears the quickest and the most completely when people die. Let's not do the job half way. Help me carry her to your bed.

ELECTRA: Did you hear her? Did you hear what my mother thought of Electra? Is it true? Did she lie?

PYLADES: I'm even less interested in your purity than in your beauty, scrupulous Electra. But I'm counting on your courage. Stop trembling like a woman or like a leaf. Take this package by its feet.

ELECTRA: Let me catch my breath. She is too heavy. She is heavy and flabby. She is slack, dead weight; it is like carrying sand or dough. And her nose is bleeding. Call Orestes!

PYLADES: Put this handkerchief over her face. Try to spare your brother this Punch and Judy show of death.

SCENE 3

Electra, Pylades, Orestes.

ORESTES: Is it over? Everything's over. I don't see any blood. But Electra's face has aged. Electra, is my mother gone?

ELECTRA: Don't worry, Orestes. Your mother bled less than at your birth, and probably suffered less also.

ORESTES: I didn't hear anything but two women's voices so alike, that it was as if Electra was insulting herself. I stopped my ears at the first cry but I could still hear the noise.

ELECTRA: The words, you did not hear the words? You did not hear what she was yelling at me, Orestes?

ORESTES: Nothing but a sound of voices, like the sound of a quarrel I once heard in a Pylos brothel. That's all my mother's death amounted to.

PYLADES: And what was your mother but the madam of that brothel?

ORESTES: I come from this body that is already beginning to rot. And once a man loved her enough to conceive me in her, in this horrible mass. I can't disown her without disowning half of Orestes.

PYLADES: The formless child you're speaking of was not this grown Orestes, changed and already destroyed by eighteen years of experience. And life had not yet turned this woman into a sick ogress. You never met this creature before.

ELECTRA: She broke in my hands like a watch. I squeezed for a minute and she got away from my grasp.

PYLADES: Fluff this pillow; fold this bedspread. Let's make her look like a heap of blankets on this bed after a bad night. The play has just begun.

ELECTRA: I couldn't go on. I have played my part.

PYLADES: Indeed, now it's the men's turn, and now you are just a walk-on. Do you hear these voices at the bottom of the hill? As expected, he is leaving his guards at the entrance of the garden. Open the door for him, Electra. Be the smiling hostess welcoming him on the threshold. I'll manage to bolt the door behind him without his noticing it.

ELECTRA: Me, smile at him with this face?

PYLADES: It won't be your first lie. Are the actors all in their places? Is everything clear? One, two, silence.

SCENE 4

Electra, Pylades, Orestes, Aegisthus.

AEGISTHUS: (*Outside.*) Electra! Is this Electra's house?

PYLADES: Go on, girl! Faster. No pity for your mother's seducer.

ELECTRA: (*Pulling the door ajar.*) Electra here. Clytemnestra's daughter, Aegisthus' stepdaughter.

AEGISTHUS: In five years you haven't learned yet how to smile, Electra. Where's your mother?

ELECTRA: My mother is resting. I forced her . . . I made her rest.

AEGISTHUS: Are you alone together? Who is this man by the hearth? Electra's husband?

PYLADES: Only an ally. Electra's ally.

AEGISTHUS: It's you Pylades? What are you plotting here? Are you playing the go-between in a reconciliation?

PYLADES: No, at a conclusion, Aegisthus. I'm helping Electra to conclude today.

AEGISTHUS: And who's this young man hiding his face with his two hands? I won't stand for masks even if they're only two bare hands. Let's see your face, my boy. What, Orestes?

ELECTRA: How can you recognize him? You haven't seen him since he was a schoolboy in knee pants.

PYLADES: The woman Aegisthus seduced was no longer young. What he recognizes, in this pure oval face framed by blond curls, is a lover he never possessed, an eighteen-year-old Clytemnestra.

AEGISTHUS: Dear Pylades! You brought Orestes back to his mother. She saw Orestes again. Where is your mother?

PYLADES: This is the last scene, Aegisthus. The playwright gathers his characters together and the curtain is about to fall. If by chance the playwright is God, his melodrama deserves only the cat calls of the audience.

ELECTRA: There is no audience here, Pylades. No one but Electra will ever see Electra's drama.

AEGISTHUS: Where is your mother? I gave in to her whim, I allowed her to visit this maniac. What have you done with your mother, Electra?

ELECTRA: I took her back. I gave her back to her son. The monster who terrified me is dead, as is the divided, unpredictable, incomprehensible creature; the woman torn between her husband and her lover, between us and you, is whole now, uncomplicated. She doesn't try to justify herself anymore, she doesn't accuse herself anymore. She is quiet. Do you recognize her? You watched her sleep so often. The Clytemnestra resting here is no longer yours, she belongs to us, her children. We are the only thing about her that, at this moment, links her to reality. Ah, Pylades, now I understand that my fake pregnancy was nothing more than a clumsy effort to match her fecundity. And don't say that I didn't treat her well, Aegisthus. Look, the marks of my fingers on her neck are almost gone, and the puffiness in her face is going down; my mother is almost beautiful again.

AEGISTHUS: Poor Clytemnestra! She left this morning in such a good mood. She was so happy to play the grandmother preparing the arrival of her first grandson. You used your child to kill your mother.

ELECTRA: Do you think me so low that I would let a peasant make love to me? Electra is still a virgin.

PYLADES: Insignificant point, Electra. Aegisthus has never been interested in your virginity.

ELECTRA: What! No tears! Yet you loved her. You loved your wife, your queen? Let's see you make a face. The paramour doesn't even mourn his old mistress?

AEGISTHUS: Your mother, Electra, has been sick now for two years with a fatal illness. You spared her a few months of suffering.

ELECTRA: She would have died surrounded by the best physicians, nursed by you till the end. She was scared; I made her suffer.

AEGISTHUS: If it's me you wish to torment, you're losing your time, Clytemnestra's daughter. I've resigned myself, a long time ago, to the idea that all will end badly, that the maniacs will win out, and that the guiltless will go down in history as murderers.

ELECTRA: Oh, you find your accomplice guiltless, do you? This guiltless woman committed not only adultery but murder as well, and furthermore she cheated on you too, now and then, with servants or hunting guests. Because, she was not faithful to you either, Aegisthus. She told me so. Confessions are easy between women. You were as cuckold as my father.

AEGISTHUS: I never begrudged my wife her little pleasures and diversions. She wouldn't have been the tender, lively creature I loved if she could have resisted squeezing, under the table, the knees of the young navy officers, or flirting with handsome boys in barley fields. Poor woman, she lied so little. Each of her naive whims moved me like the sight of a gaudy jewel she wore on her already sagging breasts—it was proof that my Clytemnestra was still

Clytemnestra. You have yet to learn that to a couple reaching our age, indulgence comes as naturally as quarrels or delights. You have not killed the woman I loved: my attachment to Clytemnestra was no longer measured by the standards of silly love. What you destroyed was a certain way of breakfasting together, a certain type of business conversation, or card playing spats, the taste of certain dishes which I ate because she favored them, the fancy for certain walks she took with me to humor me and that I shall never take again without her. In other words, half of my life.

ELECTRA: Fine. Soon, the second half of your life is going to join the first.

AEGISTHUS: You don't have to tell me. I'm forty-eight years old and I don't envy those who are sixty. At the most, there's about fifteen years left to manage Orestes' estate, and to teach him about state business. You'll never know, Electra, how much your mother loved that son you managed to deprive her of. No matter what horrible death you gave her, I forgive you if you gave her back Orestes for one second before she expired.

ELECTRA: Do you think I would let Orestes dirty his hands on the neck of women? She died alone without knowing that her son was within earshot, alone with me, her Death. We saved Orestes for the men's turn.

PYLADES: Stop dividing your attention between a dead woman and a living one, Prince Aegisthus. Orestes is in a hurry to go back to Argos tonight. Your tutelage won't be able to last more than a half-hour.

AEGISTHUS: So Clytemnestra's death was not just the result of a scuffle between two women trying to tear each other's eyes out. The soldier of fortune and the old maid planned the classic ambush together with gags for victims, sacks for two corpses, quicklime in the cellar, and an escape door opening on the gulf. Were you their accomplice, Orestes, my son?

ELECTRA: Orestes doesn't have to answer to you. He'll only have the right to speak up when his mother's lover will have disappeared.

AEGISTHUS: After having reproached me the use of my police so many times, you neglect to take into account your enemy's habits. This shanty is surrounded by my guards. I was crazy enough to entrust a mother to the natural feelings of a daughter. Believe me, I didn't have the same sense of security for myself, especially where Electra is concerned.

ELECTRA: These walls are too thick for you to be able to alert your guards. Let's say that these stones and this mortar were my mother's and your excuse for not hearing me weep. Call out, and you, yourself, will have given us the signal for your death like a man facing the execution squad giving the order to shoot.

AEGISTHUS: And what do you have to say, Pylades? Of the whole group surrounding Orestes you were the most useful being the most corruptible. Should I have doubled your subsidies? Is that the advice you gave Orestes?

ELECTRA: Say that again, very slowly, so that I can understand. Pylades was on your payroll? You knew where my brother was hiding?

AEGISTHUS: You only have yourself to blame, Electra, for forcing me to hire your doubtful friend. You put your brother in his hands; I would not have put my son there. Seeing that you entrusted Orestes to Pylades, the black sheep of his family, I had no choice but to make him my go-between, the only secret agent possible between Orestes and me, the only counsellor who might have brought him to eventually reject your lies, to choose his mother's tenderness over his sister's wrath. On this last point Pylades duped me; he's even incapable of honest betrayal.

ORESTES: So my friend was just one more cog in the horrible machine, one of the panels of the mirror reflecting Aegisthus and my mother? That clean bond of common misfortune wasn't even clean. The solitude of exile wasn't even solitary. I was only a child taken from one cage to another.

PYLADES: How could we have made it otherwise, Orestes? What harm was there in my extracting from him the money you were entitled to? Have you forgotten that princes in exile are forced to display a princely poverty? Especially you; I can't really picture you poor.

ORESTES: Why then work me up against him if our plans for vengeance already contained this portion of acquiescence? Am I going to live out my whole life in a world where every mined corridor leads to another deep one, where every secret hides a secret, where every lie conceals another lie? If Pylades was on Aegisthus' payroll, why was he readying his death?

PYLADES: Maybe for that very reason, Orestes. So that I could forget and you would not know that I could be bought.

ORESTES: But why take his money? Don't you realize that, willingly or not, I am your accomplice and that it was me this man was buying?

PYLADES: I thought I explained it to you. Because my solitude had friendship as goal and limitation. Because the brother and sister are the only friends in the world I have. Because I loved you.

ORESTES: If only I knew if you lied to him to serve us, or if you alternately served and betrayed us. Am I condemned to live forever among creatures who change form?

PYLADES: At first I thought about the profit I would make from this reconciliation between exiled stepson and rich stepfather. Then hatred for this man who employed me, precisely because he was employing me, turned me against him. Do you really need many reasons to hate someone? Your Aegisthus disgusts me. He's a man fed, protected, covered by women—a man of the world, an adventurer who made good, a sly conniver who has only one black mark against him, and who has committed, with all due precautions, only one crime. Little by little, the brother and sister dragged me into their whirlwind; I no longer distinguished between sweetness and fury. Orestes' gaze; Electra's face.

AEGISTHUS: Don't make me laugh in front of the dead. You're not in love with Electra?

ELECTRA: And why wouldn't he be in love with me? You're in love with my mother.

AEGISTHUS: Do you know men so little, Clytemnestra's daughter? But, all in all, only an innocent or a lecher can love Electra. You're in a fine mess between the fancier of young men and the gardener's helper.

PYLADES: Your own knowledge of people is singularly lacking, Aegisthus. You ought to know that any clear-headed man ends up one day by loving only Electra.

ORESTES: And all this happened around me without my knowing it! Almost without my knowing it! I'm like a man who suddenly discovers monsters living in his water glass. Electra loves me, not only as a sister, but as the mother whose place she took. Electra presented me the love of Electra like a law from which all laws derive. She loved in me the potential Orestes, the one who would satisfy her ambitions and justify her revenge; she loves me enough to save me or to break me. No, no, I'm not accusing you, unfortunate sister. If there still exists in me a sort of continuity, if there is still something hard and solid, like a stake or post, in my universe, it's Electra's love. And granted, Pylades loved me. He loved me enough to sink into God knows what vile and dangerous plotting for me, and besides, his mind enjoyed the calculation and concentration of the game. And in this confusing world I grope around in, I don't even wonder anymore if he loves the brother of Electra in Orestes, or if he loves the sister of Orestes in Electra. But you, Aegisthus, you the enemy, you the outsider. I fled my mother's house to escape death, the death of a son which would have left you the sole owner of everything. I fled Aegisthus. And meanwhile you knew where I was, you knew the names I was hiding under. You secretly dispensed the bread you could have easily poisoned. You wanted me to live.

AEGISTHUS: And why would I have wanted you to die?

ORESTES: You supported, paid for this life that was plotting your death. Those expensive rings, those horses, those race dogs, those extravagances of friend to friend, they were your extravagances, your folly, maybe your affection.

ELECTRA: He was trying to corrupt you through an intermediary. He knows the power of money, the potency of happiness. He almost succeeded in putting you to sleep.

AEGISTHUS: You didn't leave me the choice of means, Electra. My only mistake was not making of Pylades a confidant, as well as an accomplice. I should have told him the one last truth, this unique secret that would have put him uncontestably on Aegisthus' side.

PYLADES: I think I can guess this unique secret. It's not as important as you think.

ORESTES: No, Electra. I will accept neither this benevolence nor this one removed corruption. You only corrupt those you fear. And certainly he did not fear me. Or those you love.

AEGISTHUS: The time has come then to use this ridiculous word full of implications and misunderstandings. I love you, Orestes. Don't be mistaken on the meaning of this affirmation, Pylades, and you, Electra, think back and ask yourself when I first met your mother.

ELECTRA: Liar! I remember your first visit to the castle. She had made me wear a white dress with a blue bow, and I refused to greet the stranger. Orestes was a baby in the cradle.

AEGISTHUS: You have the wrong dates as far as your mother's love life is concerned, obtuse Electra. Orestes' birth decided Clytemnestra to introduce me in the household to get the servants and her other children used to me. But I have older, freer memories. I remember a young neglected wife meeting a cousin of her husband on a deserted beach, on a dry and pure summer day. I remember assignations in the woods where tree branches shielded the couple like night or twilight, and the woman yielding, as though to sleep, by a fountain. I remember meetings in the forest-ranger's house on evenings where the beloved used the pretext of going to church or the nursing of a sick farm wife as an excuse to go out; I still picture the faded cover of a peasant's bed, the dry twigs burning in a hearth, the squeaking of pine trees bent by night and the wind. Ah, I could almost tell you by what creaking of branches, by what moon ray slowly crossing the face of the sleeping woman, by what nocturnal bird call Orestes was conceived.

ORESTES: So that I am the product of this betrayal, of the lie! So that their kisses concern me more than the renown of the other man, Agamemnon. So that I've cried for the wrong father since the age of twelve.

ELECTRA: He's lying! Stop up your ears, Orestes. Can't you see that he's lying because he doesn't want to die.

PYLADES: Choose, my friend. One chooses one's father more often than you think. Choose which of the two you'd rather hate.

AEGISTHUS: Orestes explained my life and that of the unfortunate woman you have just killed. He justified the murder of a husband who refused to miscount lunar cycles. Didn't we have to act right away, as soon as he returned, so that he could not heed the servants' gossip; what else did we do but save our child? And don't tell me, Electra, that you hadn't guessed such an obvious secret. You, the spy, you the little stool-pigeon, don't tell me that you didn't know why your mother was so fond of her lastborn. The truth is we would not have been in such a hurry if Clytemnestra hadn't been afraid Electra would denounce us. All your efforts to infect Orestes with your hatred, to separate him from us makes sense only if you knew with what refinements you avenged adultery, and that the child you took from us was our child.

ELECTRA: If that's the truth, what stopped you from screaming it and driving me from Orestes' heart like an idiot who didn't understand?

AEGISTHUS: Did I have the right to dishonor my son, to annul his titles, his chances to endure after me? The greatest proof of love possible to Orestes was to hide him from his father.

ELECTRA: What he says seems to make sense. A judge would weigh his story against mine and wouldn't be able to decide which one is heavier in lies, and no one can distinguish between the son of the offender and the son of the offended. No, not even through a physical likeness since Orestes looks like my mother. Not only did they kill my father, but they also killed my brother after letting me believe that I had a brother. And I held the product of a crime between my arms. Therefore one simple truth added or suppressed can change everything. I might as well have wished to kill Orestes, that intruder.

PYLADES: So here is another lie you made your mother pay for.

ELECTRA: Not the slightest suspicion, not the slightest mistrust within me. Or did I really suspect without knowing it? So that I, the so-called loyal daughter was really kidnapping the adulteress' son. Was I getting even with Orestes' father? Ah, my brother, I loved you as a son—did envy, jealousy, deep hatred explain my maternal love? Could Clytemnestra have been right?

PYLADES: Quiet, girl. Hold fast to yourself, Electra, as to a mast. It's always easy to put things into question.

ELECTRA: Are they siding with each other against me already? Have they decided to punish the mad woman? How dim the first murder seems! Electra, the daughter of a forgotten man!

AEGISTHUS: Take your sweetheart away, Pylades; reassure her since you love her. You can leave her safely. I'll explain Clytemnestra's death by inventing a heart attack. There's been enough blood and noise around Orestes.

PYLADES: We missed our chance. Come, Electra. There's always still the world and a ship.

ORESTES: Where are they going? I don't understand. Have they stopped loving Orestes?

AEGISTHUS: Let them go, as unsure and pathetic in their wandering as two blind people in broad daylight. For us, my child, the sun has risen. We mourn your mother, but the absence of the mother simplifies the dealings between father and son. You have left now the world of women and their accomplices, the world of false friends and half sisters. But to be cautious, we won't tell this secret that makes me your roots and you my issue. Like all great loves, our love will remain hidden. I'll induct you into a world of facts and gold, of precision and solidity. I will teach you everything I know, I'll try to spare you everything I have suffered. Aegisthus' son will justify my life.

ORESTES: Aegisthus' son! For eighteen years I was the son of the other one, the murdered one, the redbearded man who was slaughtered upon his return home. How I hated him, the father who forced me to avenge him! I staggered under the task like a young soldier carrying the weight of a dead general away from the battlefield. And now suddenly I'm Aegisthus' son. Now I'm forced to resemble someone else, not only to resemble him, but to tolerate him, not only to tolerate him but to support him, maybe even to console him. This man is what I'll look like in twenty years. And I'll have to carry his history, I'll be stuck with his memories. I, Orestes, will never get out of this mess.

AEGISTHUS: You don't even have to love me. I'm perfectly content to love you as myself.

ORESTES: Let me go. Don't hang around my neck, don't look at me with that look that says you'll put up with anything because I am your son. Take that and that! I never thought I would be so glad to strike you!

AEGISTHUS: (*Stumbling.*) What have you done? This knife . . . My god! My poor child.

PYLADES: (*From the threshold.*) Come, Orestes. One never knows in this world whether one is the avenger of his father, or a patricide.

ORESTES: Electra. Give me your arm, Electra. The arm I've gotten so used to. Don't leave without me. Don't climb into the ship without me. Now we're alone. Now the three of us are alone in the world.

ELECTRA: Let's leave before night, before the sea does . . . But what's Aegisthus doing? He's turning around. He's looking at us with a look that is no longer of this world. He's trying to put a whistle to his lips. He'll manage to have us killed before he dies.

PYLADES: We'll get out of here, come what may. Orestes, come.

SCENE 5

Electra, Pylades, Orestes, Aegisthus, then the guards.

(*The guards alerted by Aegisthus' whistle appear on the threshold and on the entry to the corridor simultaneously blocking both exits. Aegisthus gestures for them to move away.*)

AEGISTHUS: Let these two men and this woman leave in peace. They are going to the shore. I told you to let them go in peace.

PYLADES: Come, Electra, and you, Orestes, don't feel too sorry for your victim. You'll have the rest of your life to decide if you should thank Aegisthus for this act of clemency. Come. The way through the pineforest is the shortest.

ORESTES: Now we are tied together. Now we're alone. Now we are free. Hold me up. Come. A sister's shoulder, a friend's arm. I am Electra's brother.

(*They leave together. Disconcerted the guards go up to Aegisthus.*)

SCENE 6

Aegisthus, the Guards, then Theodore.

AEGISTHUS: (*To the guards.*) Hold me up. I've just been wounded by some high-way men. You'll tell everyone that I was wounded by masked highway men. Highway men who fled. Those two men and that woman were innocent; they wore no masks. That's it, put me on that bed.

FIRST GUARD: (*Going up to the bed.*) Careful. Easy does it. My God, the Queen!

AEGISTHUS: The queen was wounded before me. Go fetch me a glass of water in the kitchen.

SECOND GUARD: (*To the first.*) How pale he is. Do you think we should call a doctor?

AEGISTHUS: No, no doctor. And as little commotion as possible. Here I am lying next to Clytemnestra. Come here guard. Do you hear me? You don't really understand what I'm saying but it doesn't matter, as long as you don't forget it. Don't forget to repeat later that I upheld, till the end, Orestes' rights, Orestes' candidature. Orestes. Understood?

FIRST GUARD: My Lord.

(*The third and fourth guards come in dragging behind them a dazed Theodore all tied up, his arms still full of packages.*)

THIRD GUARD: We arrested this man just as he was sneaking into the kitchen. He says he knows nothing. He pretends to know nothing. He's not wearing a mask but maybe he's one of the accomplices?

AEGISTHUS: Let him approach. Closer. Oh, it's you Theodore, the gardener's helper! Your house has become a morgue in your absence.

THEODORE: God had the lamb strike down the lion. By what miracle, Lord? Did they risk their lives while Theodore was out? Was Electra preparing for death the morning she kissed me?

AEGISTHUS: Your Electra is sailing on the sea with her lover. She has forgotten that a Theodore ever existed.

THEODORE: Thank you celestial powers for saving Electra! And I forgive you for having made Theodore the useless player who comes bearing flour and sugar when it is all over.

FIRST GUARD: What do you want us to do with this man, My Lord?

AEGISTHUS: Let him go. He's only a poor idiot. Ah, my head is spinning. Dying is nothing, what's hard is leaving life behind.

SECOND GUARD: How pale he is! How pinched his lips are! By God, Princes die like anybody else.

FIRST GUARD: It's over. He's dead as a doornail. What a mess we're in with that story.

SECOND GUARD: You really think he's gone?

FIRST GUARD: Look at him. He's not faking. Nothing could be deader.

THIRD GUARD: If we made sure that that man here . . . We've got to hold somebody.

FIRST GUARD: Well, my boy. Let's see if you can explain your presence at the scene of the crime. It's not enough to look idiotic to be innocent.

THEODORE: Let's go then. Show me the way. No handcuffs, I'll go unfettered. The victims have killed the tyrant. The angels have accomplished their butcher's task. You are right. I know everything. Nothing occurred without me. I am Electra's husband.

END

To Each His Minotaur

[1943]

LIST OF CHARACTERS:

Theseus
Voices:
    Voice of Theseus as a child
    Voice of Theseus as a young man
    Voice of Theseus as an old man
    Voice of Autolycos
    Voice of Antiope
    Voice of Helen as a little girl
    Voice of old Aegeus
    Voice of Laches
    Voice of Ariadne
    Voice of Phaedra
    Voice of Hippolytus

Ariadne
Phaedra
Autolycos
The King Minos
Bacchus (God)
The fourteen victims

The director who will stage this play will decide what sets, if any, should be used. I myself see, for the daylight scenes, vivid colors, and an almost total absence of forms: ochre and reddish tones for Crete, white marble and white foam, blue sky and blue sea for Naxos. For the scenes at sea, deep blue setting off a white sail (scene 3), or a black sail (scene 10). For scene 1, it might be a good idea to show only the top of the mast with the crow's nest which holds Autolycos. This crow's-nest, the prow of the ship (scenes 3 and 10), the tower (scene 4), and the labyrinth's door (scene 5) should be indicated symbolically by props without any attempts to reach archeological or other kinds of realism. As for the two scenes taking place in total darkness, for scene 2, in the hold of the ship, a big lamp hanging between decks could provide enough light; its movements back and forth will do to suggest the ship's oscillations. Scene 6 in the labyrinth could be played in the dark, offset by voices, or with spurts of light showing shadowy characters stumbling against a partially visible Theseus. As for costumes, according to the text, Theseus wears the red velvet cloak, the white plumed helmet and the golden armor of Greek heroes portrayed by baroque painters, but a simple braided uniform could do. Autolycos, the sailor, can wear the simple brown tunic of ancient slaves, or blue jeans. Minos could easily be wearing a cardboard crown. It doesn't matter if Phaedra is dressed as a Parisian or a woman from Crete, but Ariadne should probably be wearing a linen dress. As for Bacchus (God), he should, if possible, be very handsome.

SCENE 1

At the top of the mast. Autolycos, alone in the crow's-nest.

AUTOLYCOS: How blue the sky is! Nothing could be bluer! And beneath the
liquid blue of the sky, the solid, dense blue of the waves. The vessel I helped
build, (for I worked in the boatyards of Athens), is a closed world, a prison
loaded with inmates condemned to death. It advances, pushed by the wind;
it moves towards its own ship's destiny, and carries with it our human fate.
The weather was just as good the day I opened the goatskin in Ulysses' ship
and unleashed the storm. It didn't matter; I am a good swimmer. The
weather was just as fine the day I embarked with the Argonauts for a few
copper coins which, to me, were worth just as much as the Golden Fleece.
It's been five days since the purple Hymettus, the gray Parnes, and the little
goddess figure that signals Athens slipped from sight. Five days of pitching
and rolling: five days of this chaos which is for Neptune the eternal order of
things. The fourteen victims promised to the jaws of the Minotaur swear
and pray in the stinking hold of the ship, alternately jostled and gently rocked by the motion of the waves. Sublime, standing wind-blown on the prow
of the ship as though it were a throne, Theseus thinks about death perhaps
more tragically than the prisoners in the hold, for they have only to succumb while he must choose . . . He leans now, he's cold; he is covering his
legs with a pleat of his cape. How small these human gestures seem seen from
the height of my mast! Nothing is necessary but the pressure of my arm
grasping these ropes, nothing is inevitable but the angle of my neck, nothing

is eternal but this drop of rum dribbling down my chin. Sheep go docilely to their pastures and victims to their graves. And heroes? Where do heroes go? Me, an ordinary guy, a working stiff, Autolycos at your service, I'm not going anywhere, I am where I am. Sailor on a ship I did not charter, spectator to a drama that doesn't concern me, I lift my gourd to the health of the actors.

SCENE 2

In the hold of the ship. The Fourteen Victims.

FIRST VICTIM: The squall and that seasickness even worse than fear have stopped. The ship no longer pitches us against its sides. Even in this hold, in the darkness, you can feel that the sun is shining way up there.

SECOND VICTIM: A sun that we'll never see again since the victims of the Minotaur are only killed at night. Accursed sun shining on those who are not prisoners!

THIRD VICTIM: Yes. Yes. The weather is settling. The rest of the crossing will be peaceful. You get used to everything, even the darkness. There are still a few good moments left.

SECOND VICTIM: What difference does it make to prisoners condemned to death whether or not the crossing is good? One day more, two at the most, and we'll reach that other, unforgiving, shore; the Minotaur has been waiting for us since the beginning of time. Each oar stroke brings us closer to Him.

THIRD VICTIM: We would gain time if the wind stopped.

FOURTH VICTIM: This pre-arranged goal is still uncertain. A new storm could rise and swallow us all.

SECOND VICTIM: Either way, it's still death!

FIFTH VICTIM: Look at me, I've never been more alive. Every fiber of this body destined to the butcher quivers with joy. From time to time, a perfumed breeze penetrates the stench of this hold. And I'm holding hands with a beloved victim who, like me, will die, and with whom it will be sweet to perish.

SIXTH VICTIM: Love, it's for you I cry. Why did we meet in this wave-beaten darkness? Now I will die twice.

SECOND VICTIM: I spit upon you all, human pleasures offered in the shadows; the sensuous touch of hair brushing against my skin, the temptation of open arms. You're as repulsive as myself, future corpses, o my perishable lovers!

SEVENTH VICTIM: I think of no one but Him. Perhaps His wrath is only a sort of trial for me. And my anguish due only to my indignity.

EIGHTH VICTIM: I am sure He loves me. His hunger will devour only the guilty and the worthless. Ever since I was a child, my mother has always told me about the goodness of God.

SECOND VICTIM: And where is your mother?

EIGHTH VICTIM: No longer with us. She was picked to leave on one of the earlier trips.

NINTH VICTIM: We were chosen, one by one. We are the elected. How wonderful it is!

TENTH VICTIM: Our sacrifice saves them all. The State could not exist without us.

SEVENTH VICTIM: Such a massacre must have a reason. Let's not judge Him: let's be quiet, we who have been judged!

SECOND VICTIM: A knife! A rope! I can't stand this slow death before death! God can do nothing more to me than I can do to myself. Stab, stab, I'm carving out my red exit door. Free, at last! I foiled God's plan.

(The victim falls.)

FIRST VICTIM: What's he doing? Quick, tie his hands. He's gone crazy. He wants to die!

SEVENTH VICTIM: Too late! The poor wretch just yielded to despair. The Minotaur will not forgive him for having taken the Minotaur's place.

THIRD VICTIM: Call for help! Get the guards! Have him thrown overboard. I am scared of the dead.

ELEVENTH VICTIM: Will you idiots shut up? What's the matter with them howling like that? We're minding our own business here, playing cards in our little corner. It's so much easier to pretend that He does not exist.

TWELFTH VICTIM: If the trip lasts long enough, I could finish my poem.

THIRTEENTH VICTIM: And I, my calculation of the frequency of the waves.

EIGHTH VICTIM: If He didn't love us He would not have sent for us.

SEVENTH VICTIM: His will be done!

TENTH VICTIM: Our compatriots will remember us forever. We'll be immortal!

FOURTEENTH VICTIM: We will rot and be forgotten.

NINTH VICTIM: He tore us away from the baseness of our work-benches and shops, from the vulgarity of the sun, from the platitudes of happiness. Blessed be Thy name, Bull of the Armies!

SEVENTH VICTIM: O deadly agonies of fear! His dark breath makes my hair stand on end. God who kills us, come to our help!

FIRST VICTIM: He will trample us under his dark hoofs of ice. His horns are like the conical shadows cast by moving planets. Star dust drifts in his eyes.

EIGHTH VICTIM: He will recognize His own.

SEVENTH VICTIM: Our hearts are full of anguish, o Lord, until they come to rest in Thee.

SCENE 3

On deck. Theseus, Autolycos.

THESEUS: How moving!

AUTOLYCOS: It's only their ravings. It's not worth listening to.

THESEUS: Do they always carry on like this? Do they always weep the same hymns? Answer, o pilot of many vessels.

AUTOLYCOS: They all stammer away about God knows what. Who has time to listen to them? We're too busy tightening the ropes. A wave curls, the wind shifts, a reef upsets our keel. My duty is to see to it that the cargo reaches its port intact. For the time being, at least, they mustn't die.

THESEUS: I hear that one of them killed himself. Now there are only thirteen. Who will be number fourteen?

AUTOLYCOS: In any case, not you, young Theseus. You're much too fond of life to rub shoulders with the Minotaur.

THESEUS: Don't call me Theseus. This common name, (who knows how many people in Athens are called Theseus?) this name I have dragged with me out of swaddling clothes, then out of school and out of books, and finally out of the life my father chose for me, this name is so devoid of glory that I can hardly believe it is mine; it's always on my lips like an empty bladder I must blow up with my breath. And to no avail. Right now, my name is still anonymous. When I think that some men have the good luck to be called Hercules or Bonaparte . . .

AUTOLYCOS: Careful!

THESEUS: Why? Aren't we on the Mediterranean of all times? But the fate of the men I'm talking about is as new, as independent of the routine of history as is the light of a meteor from the seasonal migrations of the stars. As for me, I'm bound by the oaths that a Crown Prince must honor; I am entangled in secret clauses of the peace treaties. My father agreed to pay this tribute, to offer these victims to Death. He must, after all, know what he is doing.

AUTOLYCOS: I knew some cowherds from Anatolia whose job it was to transport livestock to the slaughterhouses of Athens. The animals were disembarked, tongues hanging out, emaciated by heat and by lack of water, cadaverous or half done in by beatings even before they met the clubs or knives of butchers. These people did their useful job of procuring for slaughterhouses cheaper than you do, my Prince.

THESEUS: Do you think I would have accepted this dirty job if I didn't see in it a chance for glory, a reason for being, a risk to run? I have plans like everybody else. I felt I was born to eliminate the Minotaur.

AUTOLYCOS: You felt? It seems as though I see you less often lately on the gangway consulting the stars, and half unsheathing an archangel's sword. I've seen resolves other than yours weaken during these crossings. Did the smell rising from these stacks of bodies make you quell your zeal for the job of savior?

THESEUS: I've listened to the voices in the hold too long. These victims, these martyrs: when I left, I intended to save them. But is it my place to do so? Do I have to prevent people from running to their danger?

AUTOLYCOS: They didn't choose the Minotaur.

THESEUS: They have accepted it. The Minotaur fills their soul and the ideas they have about the world; they see nothing anymore but this huge hunger as the goal of their existence. Now it's no longer the monster we have to fight but themselves. Fight to keep them on board? Hold them back, so that I can come into my own? Maybe I'm blocking their only exit toward greatness.

AUTOLYCOS: The jaws of the monster?

THESEUS: And for those who will follow. For the sacred victims yet to come. Once the Minotaur is killed, what will be left for those who wish to die? Kill Him, fine, but only so that He can be reborn. Let there be enough monsters to call forth heroes, and enough heroes to get rid of monsters until the end of time.

AUTOLYCOS: I no longer follow you very well, but I do think you're afraid.

THESEUS: Do I have the right to prefer these victims to the peace of two nations? My role as ambassador immolating his scruples is perhaps as moving as their sacrifice.

AUTOLYCOS: Don't expect me to answer. If people like me are content with subordinate positions in life, it's because they prefer leaving the honor of responsibilities to people like you.

THESEUS: If only I could be sure to have understood the wishes of my people correctly! I have asked the oracles, but in vain. Delphi ordered me to do what was right as if that was crystal clear; Trophonios advises me to be myself, as if I knew who I am. My father, when he gave me those orders, seemed tacitly to grant me leave to go against them; a defeated monarch, humiliated by the demands of Crete, he could always say that in my place, at my age, he would have understood his duties as admiral and as Crown Prince differently. How anxiously I looked at all those people the day of departure; custom guards, dock workers, money changers, shoe shiners. And this merchant's face leaning over a cold drink in a cafe of the port, and this pug-nosed ship boy's face staring at me from a launch that our ship was slowly overtaking. All of them, even the most inept ones, left it up to me to confirm, or deny, their indignity. Yet, they reserved the right to blame me for bringing war or peace, for delivering the victims or saving them. Ah, those budding girls crowned with the flowers of the land we were leaving; those groups of young men slightly paler than those groups of children riding off to summer camps, and this choir of frenzied parents, tired already of sobbing out loud. And on the neck of the youngest victim, the senile tears of my father, Aegeus.

AUTOLYCOS: Those tears that let them go.

THESEUS: Everyone is always unfair about his father; no one knew him young. Where is my father's youth? In his days, he, too, slew monsters whose skins serve now as rugs on his bed. I left to get away from him. Who could bear to see himself beforehand as a man of sixty?

AUTOLYCOS: What glory for him if you destroy the monster! But if you succumb, what a sacrifice! And if you return, an obedient son, an officer who only followed instructions, and if you have, in the pocket of your uniform, the confirmation of a good peace treaty, what glorious speeches will celebrate your precocious Statesman's wisdom! He will be sure to be re-elected president of Athens for the rest of his life.

THESEUS: That's what worries me. Docile or rebellious, I play into the hands of my family. What if I looked for a third way out?

AUTOLYCOS: There's never more than a path to the right and one to the left, Prince Theseus.

THESEUS: And what did my youth bring me except meager soldierly exploits in the colonies, and amorous conquests in garrisoned or conquered towns? Young Helen (and the little slut left with my necklace as a salary): and the Amazon, that tough blond I had to send back to her own country when I tired of the hateful wrestling she called love. And my son, a sulking adolescent who is beginning to look like his mother whom I would prefer to forget. Everything, be it pleasure or pain, was chosen for me in advance. From my father to my son, I feel like a useless link in a chain. As you see me, Autolycos, I, your prince, have also often dreamed of dark doors ajar.

AUTOLYCOS: Between the role of savior and that of butcher's accomplice, all I see left for you is the unsavory position of the victim. You were not cut out to fill the shoes of a number fourteen, son of Aegeus.

THESEUS: If only I could escape, once and for all, the destiny of Theseus, this flaccid Theseus I could become! Forswear the weariness brought on by hypothetical victories! To find, in losing, a certitude that winning lacks. What I wouldn't give to be devoured by this monstrous death after this short crossing that would then be my whole life! Yes, to perish with these young men and women . . . Instead of saving them, dying with them! To die with that tanned and warm gypsy, beautiful poppy on the side of the road, lowest of the low, picked up with those who lacked identity papers—their lot did not move the press. To die with this young Hebrew so sickly pale, so livid you want to grant him a few more days in the sun. But it's not possible. The blood that runs through my veins is not the blood of a victim; the face the mirror gives back is not the face of a victim. The only way I can matter in their lives is to save them. Ah, I'm not saying that to destroy wouldn't have been a more intoxicating and final act: there is something I would choose over killing the Minotaur.

AUTOLYCOS: What?

THESEUS: To be the Minotaur. Speaking of that, you can't hear them screaming anymore.

AUTOLYCOS: You can't hear them anymore because you yourself are speaking. You know that the noise of crowds serves only to fill in the gaps.

THESEUS: And to think that when I embarked my duty seemed so clear to me! I had it in hand like a sword. But everything got muddled as soon as the outline of the coast disappeared. Here, in this immensity between a sea in which one could drown and a sky one cannot reach, I feel less sure of being sure. Everything vacillates; the mast with respect to the sky, the sky, with respect to the mast. Don't you find this oscillation between two waves divine?

AUTOLYCOS: Pleasant, at best. Don't forget that I am a sailor by profession.

THESEUS: Delicious uncertainties! Why not stay on board forever? Fortunately we're still far from the shore.

AUTOLYCOS: My eyes are better than yours. I can spot land. Arid ground. Yellowish walls against a brown shore. It's Crete. It could be anywhere.

THESEUS: Land. How strange; by expressing my doubts, I feel I have gotten rid of them. Of all the attitudes possible, who knows if heroism isn't the easiest one? What is more complicated than the profession of ambassador?

AUTOLYCOS: And these debates with your conscience, Prince Theseus? And peace for everyone? And the right of the victims to dispose of their own lives? But are you sure, after all, that these fourteen individuals are worth saving?

THESEUS: My conscience? I have only enough time to disembark.

VOICES OF THE VICTIMS: Land. The Minotaur's cave. What do you see up there, sentries? This galloping. These mooings as night falls. Death. Death.

THESEUS: Nightfall? It's noon.

AUTOLYCOS: Don't forget Prince, they have already left time behind.

SCENE 4

A tower on the seashore with a staircase leading to the beach. Ariadne and Phaedra are on the terrace at the top of the tower. Ariadne, Phaedra, then Theseus and Autolycos, then Minos.

PHAEDRA: Sister Ariadne, I don't see anything coming.

ARIADNE: If you keep leaning out like this, you will end up falling.

PHAEDRA: I'm just waving at the passing ships. But the fishermen and the merchants go out of their way to avoid our island. No other distractions than the arrival, now and then, of cargo ships loaded with prisoners. These long lines of wretches disembarking, neck stretched, eyes lowered, grotesque as steers who have eaten their last bit of grass. None of them notice my scarf, or my proffered smile.

ARIADNE: They are gone beyond the point where women could console them. They are as absorbed in their death as we are in our solitude.

PHAEDRA: It's not a question of consoling them. Perhaps among all those clumsy men there will be one skillful enough to escape and take Phaedra with him. But let him hurry or I am going to get old.

ARIADNE: How old are you?

PHAEDRA: Strange question for a sister. I'm seventeen, and it's at seventeen that one ages the fastest.

ARIADNE: I feel ageless. Greetings, sea breeze as youthful as I am, healthy wind dissipating the stench of death.

PHAEDRA: Your only concern is that the air inhaled by Ariadne's nostrils be pure. You're as little troubled by these victims as I am.

ARIADNE: I save them as much as I can, but I try not to be contaminated by this foul atmosphere. And I'm much too busy trying not to rave on with those who rave without wearing myself out crying, each day, with those who cry.

PHAEDRA: And to whom do you intend to dedicate this purity which you take such care to guard, while I'm trying as hard as possible to bring about the seduction of Phaedra? Your solitary virtue is as useless as my desire. Don't tell me that you are not waiting for someone.

ARIADNE: Who? Don't say that I wait but rather that I am readying myself; I'm not sure that I have the right to wait. But I won't deny that I am waiting. I feel as though I am climbing on my hopes as if they were a white marble staircase. The higher I get, the further I see, but all I see is the empty ocean. More visible with each step, I become at the same time less accessible. If my climb does not stop, the only thing left to do will be to reach God.

PHAEDRA: Aren't you tired of always looking straight into the sun? How sweet the shade of forests would be after this terrace with its blinding whiteness. I wish I were invited to the Minotaur's hunting parties.

ARIADNE: You would really devour someone?

PHAEDRA: Why not? Better that than to eat my heart out.

ARIADNE: Unsated by thousands of victims, our monstrous brother howls from dusk to dawn. Do you think you would find peace in the satisfaction of your hunger?

PHAEDRA: I only want one victim. Only one face, one mouth, one golden chest to lean against, happy or unhappy. But I know he will come, I will see that creature who calls out to me from the depths of his absence. Without him, no one would know why Phaedra ever existed. And in the tight embrace of our two bodies, no one will be able to tell if I'm swooning or biting, nor if what I'm holding is my prey or my killer.

ARIADNE: I am air and breath, and I wait for the wind to strip me clean as it sweeps the fogs from the sky.

PHAEDRA: The sea weeps in me as in the breast of sad mermaids. I want to be the wave rising, breaking, unfurling and drowning someone in its wake. Look! A sail!

ARIADNE: It's leaning and turning in order not to miss the entrance to the Black Port.

PHAEDRA: It must be the victims intended for the Minotaur. We don't get much to choose from, nothing but beasts or butchers.

ARIADNE: Look, they're coming on land. An armored man leapt off the deck in a great glitter of gold.

PHAEDRA: He sees us; he is hesitating, intimidated by solitude and the presence of unfamiliar women. His bracelets, his red coat denote a Prince. Stranger!

ARIADNE: If he is the one you think he is, he will come up of his own will.

PHAEDRA: (*Starting down the staircase.*) Still, it is always safer to go down. Down with my right foot on this step, then my left foot. I instinctively know that this man will like the movement of my thighs under the transparency of my skirt and this almost imperceptible swinging of my breasts under my golden necklaces.

THESEUS: (*On the beach.*) A woman, Autolycos, an island nymph! Let's not pass up this chance for a delicious flirtation in the middle of our great adventure, nor this moment when the destiny of man is reduced to the curve of a naked waist.

AUTOLYCOS: There are two of them, Prince. That little veiled figure up there seems also worthy of the connoisseur's glance.

PHAEDRA: (*By the foot of the tower.*) My name is Phaedra. Who are you?

THESEUS: She speaks Greek. How sweet to hear my native language from lips I thought were just going to coo at me some savage tongue.

AUTOLYCOS: This is Theseus, Prince of Athens. The exportation of amphoras, the tax levied on olives, and the slave labor of Laurion mines paid for the luxury of his bracelets, his golden buskins and the ostrich feathers of his helmet.

PHAEDRA: Perfect. We are two of a kind. Tell me about Athens.

THESEUS: What should I say, Autolycos?

AUTOLYCOS: Tell her that nothing equals the beauty of our draped magistrates and our naked conscripts, that our architectural geniuses have learned how to correct the severity of vertical lines, that love and gymnastics have reached the height of pure ideas in our land. And tell her that our masterpieces will never be as perfect nor as valued as in two thousand years.

THESEUS: I have a less sublime but sweeter image of Athens than that. I'd rather assure you, Phaedra, that our twilights are purple, our water pure, our wine flavored with resin, that our sesame seed breads have a light taste unequaled anywhere else, and that our melancholic women, crowned with shiny and complicated braids, dance at night on the seashore.

PHAEDRA: If that's the case, why don't you stay with your women in Athens savoring your wines and your ripe olives? Our god devours your young men;

our island is deadly for lovers of the easy life. Your sailors are so well acquainted with that they don't dare land here. Each year they drop anchor
out at sea—you can see their pale blue pennants waving in the distance—
and the victims, driven off in the direction of the shore by whips, have to
swim towards their awaiting death.

THESEUS: From now on your god will do without victims sprinkled with salt
water. I won't hide that I've come here to kill the Minotaur.

PHAEDRA: What, our handsome monster! He and I are of the same blood. He
was born of a woman's whim, one of my mother's mad flings. His eyes are as
big as mine but sadder, and more golden. His back is as smooth as my
shoulder.

THESEUS: You are encouraging me in my endeavor, little Phaedra. A monster
who looks like you could only tempt me.

AUTOLYCOS: Don't you recognize the sailor's whore, the classic trollop found
in every port? A little more caution, my lieutenant. Your Piraeus and
Sebastopol adventures should have put you off skirts turned up by the wind
and faces smeared with paint.

PHAEDRA: And I thought you were a Prince! Make this ill-trained servant, this
common sailor shut up. My father warned me that the Minotaur's enemies
were recruited among the scum of ports and the rabble of cities. But you are
handsome: I don't see on your arm the green or black band that would place
you among pariahs and hostages. You are as strong as one can be in a world
where the Minotaur attacks only the weak, where the misfortune of losers is
the daily fare of gods and princes. And I am here, and you come into this
garden at the time of the year when the rose replaces the jasmine. You are
the first man I want to see smile and suffer, the first I want to reject and press
against my heart. My mother told me that's how you can tell you're in love.

THESEUS: This boat contains thirteen victims whose lives I promised to save.
You wouldn't want a coward.

PHAEDRA: Even less a cripple or a corpse brought back on a litter at dawn. I
prefer the living to the heroes.

THESEUS: At this very moment, head bent, the Minotaur is charging in the
corridors of the Labyrinth. He is hungry. He feels the hour of executions
and gorgings is drawing near. Phaedra, we have a whole lifetime for pleasure
and only this night for courage. I would not be able to bear the mooings of
the monster mingled with the moans uttered with Athenian accents, or to
hear them spit out my name as they heaved their last sigh.

AUTOLYCOS: Before the conversation gets too intimate or stormy, look at this
pot-bellied character approaching on the quay, unhurriedly like a bourgeois
taking his little stroll in a sunny park. Your future father-in-law, Theseus, arrives just in time to bless the lovers holding hands, and at the precise moment that port photographers are rushing towards us.

MINOS: (Coming in.) What? Who are you? I'm not very fond of strangers.

THESEUS: I am the ambassador from Athens.

MINOS: You are a representative? That's good. I no longer need to ask who you are. Athens. Let's see. Athens' quota was fixed at fourteen hostages between the ages of eighteen and forty. Your ship probably contains the annual revenue allocated the Minotaur?

THESEUS: Fourteen helpless individuals that Athens yields to the jaws of a foreign monster with regret. Fourteen victims whose fate is in my hands, and whom a great nation agrees to deliver only out of respect for signed agreements.

MINOS: The fear of risks and the respect for signed agreements are the alpha and omega of the wisdom of nations. Like yourself, I despise these human sacrifices bloodying our island, although rumor exaggerates their number. But the mystery of the Labyrinth is too complex to allow utopists, strangers and atheists to interfere. Furthermore, the bonds that unite me to the Minotaur are incredibly complicated. In a certain sense, He and I collaborate: this cutlass sharpens the goose feather with which the laws are written. And if I dare say so, Athens overestimates the value of its merchandise; as interesting as they may be as victims, the individuals in question are probably mediocre as ordinary human beings, and rather harmful as citizens. Indignation, young man, is counter-productive in the career of an ambassador.

THESEUS: I'm only indignant in the face of the crime. I only wish that order may rule in a world without evil.

MINOS: I am pleased to see then that we agreed on the principles involved. Everything will go according to form, and more pleasurably than you would have imagined. Our cuisine is famous; our bullfights are unique in the world. My daughter will initiate you to the refinements of the capital. An auto-da-fé followed by fireworks is part of the show we put on for foreign princes.

AUTOLYCOS: It's my function to divulge things. I warn you, King Minos, that this morning my master was plotting the assassination of the Minotaur.

MINOS: Bah! Boastings of a red-blooded young man. I have faith in the solidity of walls, the ingenuity of locks, the charm of women and the prestige of Laws. Forty years of political experience have taught me that heroes very seldom shake up the security of the Government.

THESEUS: Your invitation honors me, Majesty. But who is that little veiled figure, distaff in hand, walking away without looking at us like a working woman going home at nightfall?

PHAEDRA: Ariadne, my sister. She spends her life doing good deeds. Every day, she is busy putting her little room in order.

SCENE 5

*A rocky landscape. A mountainside, a gigantic door which is closed. Autolycos,
Theseus, then Ariadne.*

AUTOLYCOS: The door is shut.

THESEUS: It must have closed on its own. What an awful night. You can't
imagine . . .

AUTOLYCOS: You forget that I was with you.

THESEUS: You can't imagine how horrible I feel for missing my chance to em-
bark for glory, and through my own fault. Bewildered as a traveler stranded
on a quay, I watch immortality sail away in the distance.

AUTOLYCOS: Regrettable for you, this negligence is a disaster for our thirteen
poor devils—supposing that those people would have preferred to live.

THESEUS: My intentions never faltered in spite of solicitations and magical
obstacles. I was determined to save those people till the very end.

AUTOLYCOS: As determined as you were to enjoy Phaedra.

THESEUS: As if a woman mattered! And after all this, I wake up, rolled, in a
cabin stinking of jasmine, the whore gone, sailors snoring on deck, and the
key to the hold, where the victims were, gone from under my pillow. Ah, I
did not foresee those invincible narcotics, nor the deepness of this drugged
sleep.

AUTOLYCOS: Yet, the sea water I poured over you woke you from that sleep.

THESEUS: Why did you limit your services to that of the perfect servant? You
were awake; you were watching; nobody tempted you. You witnessed the
abduction of the victims without lifting a finger to help them. Your cowar-
dice disgusts me even more than my own weakness.

AUTOLYCOS: Seeing that I have neither the rewards of temptation, nor those
of glory, allow me at least to keep those of neutrality. Furthermore, I am the
one who guided you along this path overhanging the abyss. Without the
support of my arm, you would not have withstood the dizziness.

THESEUS: The fog drowned out the sea—we tripped several times on this path
the victims followed with the agility of sleepwalkers. Everything happened as
if in a dream. Those idiots must have made it a point of honor to let
themselves be dragged without struggling, believing in some order from
above, as they say. What silence! Not a single scream, not even the squeaking of the door that separates the two worlds. Even their agonies are dead.
We arrive too late to witness the crime, and this massacre is already part of
History.

AUTOLYCOS: Admit that you are pleased by the presence of the irreparable.
Tomorrow, Phaedra will explain that everything is for the best in the best of
all possible Cretes.

THESEUS: Phaedra is a whore, and I am the customer who wakes up with his wallet gone. If this story gets around, I'll be the laughing stock of Athens.

AUTOLYCOS: Stay in Crete, and the laughter from Athens will only sound from a distance. Phaedra will come back to you tomorrow, repentant, soft as a rose, ready to pay for her fifteen minutes of betrayal with all sorts of endearments. The lover, the husband of Phaedra has the best chance to succeed in eventually muzzling the Minotaur. You are still at the infancy of compromises.

THESEUS: That's it, Autolycos, give your Prince his confidence back, show him that from the ashes of the hero a reformer, a moderator can arise. Tell me how once known, controlled, Phaedra can become a beautiful tool in our hands. In the first round of a game, who cares if a few pawns are lost? The sacrifice of those victims would not be totally in vain if Minos' successor . . . Many others had a false start. Maybe there is still time to become a great man.

ARIADNE: (*Enters, carrying a lamp.*) Here I am.

THESEUS: This light . . . My god, how blond she is! It's Phaedra's sister.

ARIADNE: What are you doing in this sinister place without a guide? Where are the victims?

THESEUS: (*Embarrassed.*) What victims? I was waiting for you.

ARIADNE: (*Softly.*) You are lying.

THESEUS: I was waiting for the one who would come. That's what I have been doing my whole life.

ARIADNE: And they did not come?

THESEUS: They came and went. A few, like your sister, left too soon, the soldier's meager savings tucked into their hastily gathered clothes.

ARIADNE: To each her own. My sister strives to destroy you as I would like to create you. But you chose to love Phaedra.

THESEUS: One chooses the women who offer themselves. Phaedra was the first to welcome me on the quay of a new world. Why didn't you approach me sooner, inalterable and pure figure? Your silences would have warned me, your shadow on the sand would have indicated that the hour of my life had struck. But Phaedra took from me the right to say the words that would open Ariadne's heart.

ARIADNE: I wait for a sign before I offer myself. It's by that caution that you can recognize women who are truly chaste.

THESEUS: If that's the case, who summoned you to this lair at midnight? It hadn't occurred to me to call for you from the depths of my shame.

ARIADNE: The nurse risen before dawn greets the soldier climbing towards the enemy. Later, you will measure yourself up against the Cause of all evil.

THESEUS: This deferred fight has become singularly useless. I sinned. My friends are no more.

ARIADNE: Think of the victims yet to come. It's always the same people who perish. You will save your friends from a second death.

THESEUS: How? The door is shut again; the walls are impenetrable. You can't get into Hell simply by willing it.

ARIADNE: Look at that gray crack just wide enough to let a human shoulder get through. Since I have been here the door opened again. You did not notice it.

THESEUS: Then, I might as well resign myself to heroism. It's not easy. The Labyrinth has complications worse than death, solitudes more fatal than that of combat. I am afraid of getting lost. I am not sure I won't disgrace myself.

ARIADNE: Take this thread. Its strands are more solid than the steadiest of human thought; its length is exactly that of your future steps. Whatever happens, you are tied to me like a new-born to his mother.

THESEUS: How can I express . . . I am very moved, Ariadne. Up to today, I have existed alone. Up till now, women were traps or sometimes ghosts. Men were comrades, or rivals, or enemies. Even my son . . . Even my father . . . But I don't have time to tell you about my son or my father. I'm entering the Labyrinth attached to you by an indestructible thread. I will walk towards death, sweetly committed to the future. The most banal metaphors take on new life; a fountain flows, a lamp lights up of its own in my life. Ah, I didn't foresee this happiness of having a woman . . .

ARIADNE: I am not a woman, I am yours.

THESEUS: I hardly believe in you as a woman. How I'm going to love you, my friend!

ARIADNE: The moon is setting; all you can see now in the fog is one of the horns of this white heifer. The skies are hard and dark like steel and courage. Go, my heart.

THESEUS: Stay, my soul. Autolycos, I put her in your hands. Am I cheating? It's getting almost too easy. The woman . . . The thread . . . (*He disappears.*)

ARIADNE: He's gone.

AUTOLYCOS: What spoils your part for me is that you run no risks.

ARIADNE: I risk being mistaken about him.

AUTOLYCOS: That's already done; you take him for a great man.

ARIADNE: Don't set him straight, if it's his delusion. What is a hero at first if not a poor man trembling? Perhaps there is false pride in reeling off from above the fate of a creature, but I also spare him superfluous worries. He will find himself in finding me.

AUTOLYCOS: Do you think he has met up with the Minotaur? One can't hear anything.

ARIADNE: Now that you mention it, by tying this thread to a seashell, you can hear . . .

AUTOLYCOS: Remarkable. Does that apparatus also transmit pictures?

ARIADNE: It will in a few hundred years. But nothing prevents us from getting a little ahead of our time. Right now, we could be anywhere in the course of

History.

AUTOLYCOS: May I give it a try? The pictures are jumbled; no doubt because it is dark. On the other hand, the voices are . . . I think I recognize Theseus' voice.

ARIADNE: One moment. No, right now it's the Minotaur's.

AUTOLYCOS: May I? How funny; they have the same intonation.

SCENE 6

In the Cave. Theseus, then the Voices.

THESEUS: I am losing my bearings. It's as dark here as in a cave. Nothing more fatiguing than to fight with darkness. It eliminates the outside world. I feel as though I am plunging into my own internal gloom, and the circonvolutions of the Labyrinth make me think of my bowels. Will I find the Minotaur in the middle of all this? If he does exist I'll be covered with ridicule.

VOICE OF THESEUS AS A CHILD: I have been hiding here for ages. When he walks by, I'll open the closet and boy, will he jump!

THESEUS: I think I hear someone. No, no one. I keep on measuring myself against an absence. Is emptiness the real danger? Ah, how . . . how monstrous! What I wouldn't give for a flesh and blood enemy.

VOICE OF THESEUS AS A CHILD: I plucked the bird. Dirty beast, there. Go on, croak a little. It's bleeding. Daddy brought eight wild ducks back from hunting yesterday. He has a rifle that goes pouf! What if the rifle burst, and Daddy was covered with red currant jelly . . .

THESEUS: Who is this kid climbing up my legs? Children in these evil haunts? He looks like . . . ouch!

VOICE OF THESEUS AS A CHILD: I have always felt like biting his hand. Why did he spank me so hard when I lied about the orchard pears?

THESEUS: They tasted sour, those orchard pears. I was wrong, of course. But still, you have to admit that my father was ridiculous with his pompous speeches.

VOICE OF THESEUS AS A CHILD: With his pompous speeches. And when he would butt in, trying to help me translate Greek verses . . .

THESEUS: Greek verse?

VOICE OF THESEUS AS A CHILD: Of course, Greek verses. Another useless language.

VOICE OF THESEUS AS A YOUNG MAN: Does he really think that I can get by on five thousand drachmas per month? Why, just that little party yesterday with the Gypsies alone cost . . . It would be absurd to spend less than Laches.

VOICE OF AUTOLYCOS: (*Persuasive.*) Of course, Lieutenant. A Crown Prince is entitled to a sport carriage. And if you are unfortunately obliged to incur debts . . .

THESEUS: (*Protesting.*) I paid my debts.

VOICE OF THESEUS AS A YOUNG MAN: My father paid. He likes paying my gambling debts because it humiliates me. But the usurer in Odessa was unbearable with his outrageous demands. If it hadn't been for the Scythian jewels stolen from a tomb . . .

VOICE OF AUTOLYCOS: Quiet, Master. You weren't stealing, just indulging your interest in archeology. You'll be elected to the Institute in your old age.

THESEUS: How beautiful they were on that white skin, those Scythian gold bracelets! And that hair, pure gold! Ariadne's hair. But her eyebrows touched, her little forehead frowned. A virgin, of course. A red virgin. A colonel from a regiment of Amazons. A captive who casts withering looks at my sentries. If I didn't know how to handle women . . .

VOICE OF THESEUS AS A YOUNG MAN: Where did you put her? I didn't tell you to lock her up in a damp cave, on stinking straw. Did you feed her? . . . She has had nothing to eat? Mark my words, the Athens newspapers will accuse us of mistreating our prisoners.

VOICE OF AUTOLYCOS: So what? She broke everything. What can you do with a wild woman like that? You speak Russian, Captain, have it out with that Amazon. Maybe she wants to save her own skin, like everyone else.

VOICE OF THESEUS AS A YOUNG MAN: Bring her out. I would rather let everything happen in plain view.

VOICE OF AUTOLYCOS: Out of the question. She's howling . . . she scratches and bites. She's foaming. A whole squad might not be enough to hold her down. You think I'm exaggerating. Look through this crack in the wall.

VOICE OF THESEUS AS A YOUNG MAN: I'm not in the habit of looking through keyholes.

VOICE OF AUTOLYCOS: Well, you've got to take some precautions. One can't say that she doesn't have pretty legs. You will excuse me, Captain, I'm going to lunch.

THESEUS: Phew! I don't know how I've been able to bear this man for so long. If he hadn't left me alone in this isbah with this girl . . . The language of a street hawker and the morals of a pimp.

VOICE OF THESEUS AS A YOUNG MAN: She is sobbing, stretched out on straw. Her uniform is in shreds. Her legs are shaking. And this sunlight on her blond mane . . . Are you afraid of me? No one will hurt you.

VOICE OF ANTIOPE: I am soldier. In my country, soldiers are not afraid.

VOICE OF THESEUS AS A YOUNG MAN: Why are you holding your hands behind your back? Have they been tied? Your hair is in your eyes. Let me push back your hair. Do I look like a torturer?

VOICE OF ANTIOPE: You look like an enemy. I spit on the enemy.

VOICE OF THESEUS AS A YOUNG MAN: You're really removing whatever scruples I may have, my girl. Ouch, what sharp teeth, like a wolf. Ah, the bitch. My mouth is bleeding. Take that, and that. She fell. She's not moving. She fainted. Her buttons popped. Her blood . . . Her breasts . . .

THESEUS: Any man would have done the same thing in my place. White as snow . . . Hard as marble . . . Besides, she immediately fell in love with me.

VOICE OF ANTIOPE: Where are you, Atalante, my companion? Walls, armies between us. And me, a prisoner, taken by force, me, vanquished. And at times, I hope for the arrival of Red troops setting fire to the city, and have him die in it. I will take back human form only by dint of hating him. And at other times, I love him. What would become of me if I did not love him? And if he tires of me, he'll pass me on the Laches, then Autolycos. He will be ashamed of having desired me so much that he got entangled with the enemy. Do I like him? Ah, if I didn't like him I would no longer be alive. I didn't know this avid beast, deep within me, that wants to make love. And my belly is heavy. When, from time to time at night, I secretly put on my uniform, it no longer hooks. And I lack the courage to kill this enemy inside of me. Yet, I can't go back home with a Greek bastard.

THESEUS: She was deranged. An unnatural mother, you couldn't deal with her. She didn't even want to keep her child.

VOICE OF THESEUS AS A YOUNG MAN: I behaved correctly towards her. I offered her Laches as a husband. Let her go back to her cabbage fields, her barracks, her snow bound village. Besides, she was not as beautiful in city clothes as she was in her Cossack uniform. Fortunately the old man is going to raise the child. A descendant, after all, the hope of the dynasty . . . Well, perhaps all this will relieve me of the task of having to marry a Highness.

VOICE OF AUTOLYCOS: What a pleasure to be back in the capital. There's no denying it, Captain, you're the one everyone is looking at. Naturally, the young hero, the conqueror of Crimea. Boy, does your father look like an old fogey in his ceremonial hat!

VOICE OF THESEUS AS A YOUNG MAN: During the procession? Are you sure? Are you sure terrorists are waiting by the Panathenaea passage, at the corner of Stadium and University streets? What do you want me to do about it? Change his route? When my father has an idea in his head, he sticks to it. Besides, security is a matter for the police. I can't look as though I'm always trembling.

VOICE OF THESEUS: Besides, nothing happened. Of course, with his weak heart, the noise of a bomb going off would have killed him. Even today, if by chance, some bad news . . . Out of consideration for him, I better not expose myself.

VOICE OF HELEN AS A LITTLE GIRL: He is looking at me out of the corner of his eye. How handsome he is. Closely shaven. And that gold necklace around his neck . . . Let's walk slowly. I have been told that men like it when you wiggle a little. I like that gentleman. As if I didn't know why he was looking at me like that. Olympia told me, after her encounter with the gardener's son.

VOICE OF THESEUS AS A YOUNG MAN: Not bad, that kid. What a brazen look! Her legs are all scratched by brambles. The road to Mistra? Do you know how to go to Mistra? Yes, with me it will be easier. Here take my hand. One, two, three, jump. There you go. Her skirt only reaches to mid-thigh. Are you afraid of the horse? Little kitten. And not dangerous, not at that age. I wonder if? . . . I hope the family doesn't make a scene.

VOICE OF HELEN AS A LITTLE GIRL: Now I'll also have things to tell Olympia. No, I'm not crying; I'm a big girl. If mother knew! Luckily, my skirt is not too wrinkled. He doesn't feel my fingers touching his necklace. What a beautiful stone, how shiny. Into my pocket, done. I'm expected at home. You're very nice. Yes, every day, on the road, to bring the goat to pasture.

VOICE OF THESEUS AS A YOUNG MAN: She's running through the fields without so much as a backward glance. She gave me something pleasant to remember. My necklace! The little slut took my Golden Fleece, that precious piece, a gift from Hercules, not another one like it in the world. That'll teach me to go around in full regalia.

VOICE OF OLD AEGEUS: And right now, in the midst of our election period . . . Theseus, my son, your frivolity is almost criminal. In Mistra, where our good Spartan allies live, and the daughter of people of high esteem. The security of the State, the good name of the dynasty . . . And why, dear god! Athens is full of better looking girls than that!

VOICE OF LACHES: We must get rid of the old fool for the sake of the dynasty's good name. You aren't going to let yourself be sent off to the colonies, my Lord? This absurd war . . . The ultimatum of the Cretan government . . . Of course, no coup d'etat without risks, but the army is, traditionally, on the side of crown princes.

THESEUS: I was right to resist the bad advice of Laches. One can't be without a conscience. And furthermore, you never know where it can lead you; you start by making someone abdicate and the next thing you know, you have unleashed a revolution. My feet hurt . . . I will come back from the colonies covered with glory. Light bones, skulls as polished as seashells . . . No, old nails, broken bottle ends . . . Where are the victims? All this seems part of a hatched plot. This bullfight arena without a bull is ridiculous.

VOICE OF ARIADNE: You are fighting the Cause of all evil. Your future steps . . . He will find himself in finding me.

THESEUS: Ouf! My arm is all stiff. I think that it's the thread that bothers me. But I couldn't hurt her feelings by refusing to accept her little invention. One never knows, it could come in handy. But what is the matter with women that they all throw themselves at me?

VOICE OF PHAEDRA: I'm languishing for Theseus. I'm dying for Theseus.

THESEUS: (Content.) Yes, little Phaedra is dying for me. I hold a slight grudge against her for that business of the fourteen victims heading for . . . Poor devils. Not very interesting samples of the human race. Put myself in her place. A dirty trick. A practical joke from a little girl who likes to see a train accident. Besides, she is crazy about me. She did it out of affection for me, so that I wouldn't lose face. It's clear as day; there are kisses which do not lie.

VOICE OF PHAEDRA: These eyes, so pure . . . Proud . . . Untamed . . . How young you are. I never met anyone as young as you.

THESEUS: Untamed . . . Well, well. But young? After all, thirty-eight is not yet decrepitude.

VOICE OF HIPPOLYTUS: Go away, go away! This heat, this odor, this female softness . . . And my father's wife . . . Never! Never!

VOICE OF THESEUS AS AN OLD MAN: (*Quivering, broken.*) She fought him. She told me so. Does a woman ever fight it? I remember, in my own case, Antiope. That was different; she was a Slav, an enemy. But your father's wife. Unnatural son, hypocrite. Ah, the wretch, I'll show him what's what . . . Prison, the ax . . . Like Peter the Great. But careful . . . The good name of the dynasty won't allow a king to have his own son executed. One can always arrange things so that it will look like an accident. What if by chance his horses went crazy and he cracked his skull against a rock?

VOICE OF HIPPOLYTUS: Pure as daylight . . . The bottom of my heart . . . Not to look like him, to have this obscene face later, this leer of the seducer of women. My mother forced, raped, insulted. A heroine in her own right, a warrior. And his marriage with this awful foreigner looking at me with rapacious eyes. And Ariadne abandoned.

THESEUS: Me abandon Ariadne? Never. My love. Whose voice is this? Who dares? I'll kill him!

VOICE OF THESEUS AS AN OLD MAN: I killed my own son. My only son. The hope of the dynasty. At the corner of two roads between Eleusis and Daphni. My son, bleeding. Blood on the road . . . My son, innocent. And what if she spoke the truth, what if she recanted to make me suffer even more, to make me believe that I had killed my son while he was innocent? And even if he wasn't, if he really had . . . We could have worked something out, the three of us. I would have closed my eyes. My son, dead. It's as if I killed myself at twenty. Should I flog myself in public? Confess on the village square? Let's not go too far, after all. People would laugh. I would be the butt of Athens. My son, Gentlemen, my poor child. Thank you . . . Thank you . . . I am very touched by the Senate's condolences. It was fate.

THESEUS: What is that old fool talking about? Kill your own son? It's a plot. Laches is right, it's either him or me. But what is he using as pretext, some silly story about a woman? He must mean that old wrinkled star, the outmoded darling of the nightclubs of Pera whom he married morganatically last year. The old sow probably told him that, out of spite . . . Of course, she would like nothing better . . . I would not have touched her with a ten foot pole. A woman that Daddy . . . I don't give a damn about his curse. Dirty old man. Nice to get rid of him. God, is he ugly! Look at that senile head! Here, take that on the nose! And that, right in the eye! I have wanted to break his face for a long time now. He cut his gray beard so that it will look like my blond beard. And that scar at the corner of his eye. Now, he is copying my scars. Your son, you said. My hands are bleeding. I hit him too hard. A good knife. Let's get it over with. It's either him or me, as Laches said. For the dynasty. Here, in the neck! In this dirty neck wrinkled like a turkey. Oh, God, it's as though I were the one who was dying! (*He collapses in a great crash of crumbling wood-work and broken glass.*)

SCENE 7

A swamp by the edge of the sea. Ariadne, Autolycos, Phaedra, Theseus.

AUTOLYCOS: No one. We are in a no man's land: torn posters, scrap iron. Something like fairgrounds the morning after the National Holiday.

ARIADNE: I see a body stretched out on the sand, a blond beard, a gold shoulder-belt. Quickly, Autolycos! It's Theseus. He just collapsed, crushed by the weight of the Labyrinth falling on him. He is choking, caught up in his own knots, entangled in the thread I gave him as a safe-conduct. That's it: pick up his head; cut the string that is strangling his neck. And you, Phaedra, have him breathe this flask of perfumes. Repentant sister, this morning your name is Magdalene.

AUTOLYCOS: Forgive me, Ladies. The little that remains from this Labyrinth is not very impressive. Is it against these papier-mâché walls, these screens plastered with fun-house mirrors that Theseus fought? A coward fainting looks very much like a hero succumbing. You are transforming him rather quickly into the Just crucified.

ARIADNE: Quiet, tasteless banterer. *Ecce Homo.* His lips are moving. Memory bubbles are bursting to the surface. Prophetic visions, once again, become bits of nightmares. Let his courage take the upper hand on his cowardness.

THESEUS: (*Coming to.*) Where am I?

AUTOLYCOS: You are in a world where Theseus still exists, where Ariadne never stopped existing. Any other information would be superfluous.

THESEUS: Phaedra?

AUTOLYCOS: Phaedra also continues. And me likewise, at your service. You can see that nothing is changed.

ARIADNE: The noise of an explosion led us to you after a night of praying. The collapse of the Labyrinth is a sign. What was horrible has become ugly. You have killed the Minotaur.

THESEUS: What? Of course. Let me try to see again, try to relive . . . I walked all night long in corridors full of traps. I saw monsters. Terrors . . . And the Minotaur . . .

AUTOLYCOS: Is he hideous?

THESEUS: He is invisible. I was assaulted by an army without ever seeing its general. And as I walked, I had to ward off battalions of bad angels. Step by step, I followed this formless Beast, this adversary whose strategy is one of constant retreat. I was caught in the wake of a breath that terrified and stunk like that of a wild beast. He dragged me to this beach. A motionless sea, vitreous waves . . . The Minotaur stuck to my body, not allowing room for my lungs, my heart. I hit Him with my fist, with the pommel of my sword. I was like a man locked up in a glass prison who, in order to escape, carves out a star, blow by blow. The Beast bit me. See my forehead, see my hands. I heard the glass shatter; great pits gaped underneath. But the only proof I have of the fight is this red stain.

ARIADNE: I believe you, Theseus, since real blood is flowing from your wounds, and no charm, whatsoever, can resist blood ablutions. The Minotaur is dead since you are bleeding. The reign of Evil is over since we are walking free on this land that ghosts formerly roamed. Forgive me to have doubted you enough to try to help you, to have insolently tied this useless string to your hand. Your strength alone was enough to counterbalance Evil.

AUTOLYCOS: Theseus conquered, granted, and it would be useless to recall that our victims were devoured. My advice, Prince, is to leave as quickly as possible these complicated grounds. To guard against all eventualities, I gave your sailors the order to get under way towards this beach.

THESEUS: If I wanted to survive, it was to smell again the honey scent of Ariadne's hair, to hear once more the sweet rustle of her linen dress in the wind. Will you follow me till the end of the world, you without whom I am less than myself.

ARIADNE: Until the end of life, if necessary. And wherever you wish to lead me, o Theseus.

PHAEDRA: And me? What about Phaedra? Ariadne, my sister, I know I sinned. But did not my obscene mother bring me into the world for that very purpose? Was my soul not marked, at birth, by the same black spots as grace a leopard's skin? Are you going to leave me alone in the middle of a world that was beautiful, and that you destroyed because it seemed evil to you?

ARIADNE: We will take you along, Phaedra. Let it not be said that our selfish happiness was grounded in sacrifice. Let it not be said that we set sail together towards a perfection you won't share. A new truth, an unknown god might be waiting for you amid the whiteness of Athens.

THESEUS: No, Ariadne. One night of trials was enough. I don't want a pretty snake on board my ship.

ARIADNE: What good is a victory that is not renewed every night, a choice that is not made again every morning? Phaedra depends on me for her light; I need her as my shadow. I can't abandon half of my life on the beach. I won't believe in your love for Ariadne unless you take Phaedra along.

THESEUS: Don't insist, my innocent girl. Don't mingle who knows what poisons to your pure perfumes. I know Phaedra better than you. You never saw her in love nor in betrayal.

ARIADNE: How do you know, Theseus, that Phaedra's pleasures or betrayals are not made up of Ariadne's silences, of my purity turned inside out, of my chastity closing its eyes. If Phaedra did not exist, perhaps Ariadne would be Phaedra.

AUTOLYCOS: Don't prolong this quarrel, Prince Theseus. The noise of the explosion must have been heard on the whole island. Don't forget that a hero caught by the police is nothing but a prisoner.

ARIADNE: Let's go. The wind is rising, the smell of the sea is already carrying us off. Everything beautiful is yet to come. We save our lives only by entrusting them to the waves.

THESEUS: Let's go. This little girl following you, this little bitch I once petted is of no consequence. We are at this hour of the morning that makes the night seem impossible. Who cares about a dark stain? Your whiteness dazzles me, blinds me. I never loved anyone but Ariadne.

ARIADNE: Follow us, Phaedra. And you, Autolycos, give your arm to our still staggering hero, our wounded soldier. What's that, little girl? What do you see there on the ground? What are you picking up?

PHAEDRA: Nothing important, Ariadne. A plaything . . . Look: a little rusty blade forgotten on the sand. A child's sword.

SCENE 8

A beach in Naxos. Theseus, Ariadne, then Phaedra.

THESEUS: The winds have fallen, Ariadne; it's the time of year the halcyons make their nests. We'll be here for weeks, or months, or forever.

ARIADNE: Crete was only a prison; every one of the Cyclades we visited on our way was just a port of call. But the calm that keeps us here, sails folded, on this deserted island, at the foot of this naked mountain, begins for us an endless era. Absolute happiness, perfect silence rule here like an eternal noon.

THESEUS: The island is uninhabited but not sterile. To my great surprise, I found many springs. Their water is cold but pure and fresh. The untended trees bear strange fruit, less nourishing than our own bland apples.

ARIADNE: These oblong beaches have the form of a zither. Tuned for centuries, they seem to be awaiting a song.

THESEUS: This morning while I was swimming, I found nuggets on the sand. There is enough gold here to build a Parthenon, or to pay for the war in Sicily.

ARIADNE: We will walk barefoot on this sand with no past, along these rocks with no memory. The flat sea will reflect a succession of dawns and sunsets, a procession of stars, but our inalterable destinies will change as little as the profile of the rock. No breeze will deflect the perfume rising from the lavender fields; no pain will deform our love, fixed in the sky like a great golden cloud. And what difference does it make if the wind rises, if this calm is only an interlude in the drama of a world not as wise as we ourselves? We have arrived. We are at the center. The word departure has lost its meaning; I no longer understand the word return. Each rock is a pedestal; each island that rises from the sea is as important to us as any other. Man's apprehension alone is to blame for the invention of Crete and the building of Athens.

THESEUS: Why remind me of Athens? Our stop in this island is going to cause a thousand political complications. I can't forget that I am the Crown Prince.

ARIADNE: In this solitude, I feel I am a queen. But you would probably tell me that's too easy.

THESEUS: Precisely. Just because we have simplified them doesn't mean that we have solved the problems. If we strip ourselves any barer, there will be nothing left.

ARIADNE: Do you think that I am interested in a picture postcard kind of happiness? Life is not easier here, nor are the problems less complicated on this island than elsewhere. There is Autolycos. There are your sailors. And you don't have to remind me that there is Phaedra.

THESEUS: I haven't seen her for a while. Where is she?

ARIADNE: Phaedra is always in your thoughts, and no one knows better than I that she is always in your dreams. Even right now, at this moment, I see you squint, searching out on this russet beach an amber colored body.

THESEUS: Phaedra, that flat spot at the foot of the rock, two arms and two legs stretched out, and a black coil of hair? From this distance, your sister, Ariadne, looks like a starfish.

ARIADNE: Do you think I'm blind? Autolycos showed me the mark left by two bodies on the sand, at the foot of the tree where two mouths bit into the same fruit. I am tired of smiles that hide and counterfeit kisses. I had offered you a choice between us, not a pretense.

THESEUS: If that's the case, what is the meaning of that song of love a little while ago, of that assertion of absolute happiness to which I have the humility not to aspire? I lie out of pity, you lie out of pride, Ariadne. It's on such a base that most couples build their lives.

ARIADNE: I'm trying to maintain the image of a happiness that would exist if you were the man you could be. What prevents you from being strong, from being sincere, from being pure? This perfect Theseus, whom I constantly protect from yourself, depends only on you to come into being.

THESEUS: It's precisely that image of a perfect Theseus that I escape from between the arms and legs of Phaedra. She's easy. All she expects of me are mediocre vices or virtues. If you were looking for a god, why did you pick a man?

ARIADNE: Because it's in the form of a man that most women expect to find God. Remember that you are the best I found to love, and that I was, for a while, the best you found as a friend.

THESEUS: All you were looking for was that ideal character women need to believe in in order to be able to make love, more or less, without shame. Your solicitude was like that of a flirtatious nurse at a patient's bedside. What's the point of marital intimacy if one can't be comfortable, if you can't take your girdle off, and me my breastplate? I am thirty-eight years old. My time for heroics is at an end, and Love with a capital L was never my specialty.

ARIADNE: How could what never happened be over? You did not kill the Minotaur.

THESEUS: You're not going to bring that up again? That was nothing more than a fiction invented by Athenian propaganda, a silly story in which I got involved against my better judgment. You seem too enlightened to believe in monsters.

ARIADNE: If you had killed the Minotaur would I be here wishing for the death of Phaedra, for yours and mine? We haven't left the Labyrinth. My love has become hate, my humility humiliation, my indulgence corruption. I count the kisses; I exult in my triumphs of the flesh. I laugh at your puns; I do not contradict your hunting stories. I belittle myself uselessly, hoping to make you greater in my eyes. And I can't see Phaedra sleeping on the sand, in the sun, without wanting to shove a rock on her.

THESEUS: And that's the way I like you. I prefer you, as you are now, to Phaedra. When your heart flutters like that beneath that boring white drapery, I am not so sorry to have signed my name on the dotted line in some forgotten Cyclades. Statue turned to flesh, none of Phaedra's wanton pleasures equal your broken scruples. After all, I didn't marry you to bring to my bed a school mistress, or my protectress, Athena.

ARIADNE: No. While there is still time, I am putting an end to what was for me the human adventure. I will not triumph over Phaedra by turning into Phaedra. I don't want to become, little by little, the jaded companion, getting along in years, who closes her eyes in return for bank accounts and jewels. Nor do I want to become the admirable spouse, her face drawn, her lips a tight-pinched line whose wink reveals that she really knows more than she lets on. I will not go from despair to exasperation, from exasperation to contempt. Take Phaedra; she was made for all your pleasures as well as your misfortunes. Lift anchor; leave with my sister for your Piraeus and your Acropolis, and leave me on the shore of this deserted island as in a bed too big for me where I can, at last, sleep alone.

THESEUS: You forget that we are stuck here because of this calm. You know very well that you don't risk being taken at your word very soon.

ARIADNE: You're mistaken. The wind is rising. Look: that tuft of verbena is shaking. And here is Phaedra; your fate is approaching on the thinnest pair of sandals. Each to his own Minotaur; you may not know it, but right now you are headed for danger.

PHAEDRA: (*Coming in.*) I am bored to tears! It does not take long to be weary of this tiresome marble sea. If I had known that we would be stopping here for such a long time, I would have brought along more luggage.

ARIADNE: See how you understand each other. Her wardrobe and your uniforms are the indispensable props you'll need to play out your roles of King Theseus and Queen Phaedra.

THESEUS: Phaedra, we are leaving.

PHAEDRA: And Ariadne is staying?

ARIADNE: I have arrived.

THESEUS: Ariadne, I do my best not to be cruel to women, but time is running out. If you absolutely insist on spending the summer on this island, far be it from me to object. Besides, the place is not as isolated as you would think. Fishing boats could . . . Well, do as you like. I did what I could to love you.

PHAEDRA: It's not my fault, Ariadne.

ARIADNE: It's mine, Phaedra. All this has been planned ahead of time. I am sorry to cause you remorse.

PHAEDRA: I don't have any. I am incapable of it.

ARIADNE: But it will get you, Phaedra. Remember me as late as possible. And give Theseus enough joy to make up for his future misfortunes.

PHAEDRA: What do you mean? He doesn't appeal to me, with that womanizer's coarse laugh. He's not young enough. Then there's that son . . . But he must have been handsome at twenty. And he is the very first one to have noticed little Phaedra. And I'm not one to settle for a second place. Well, I think I like him just enough to force him to betray Ariadne.

ARIADNE: Enough to betray me, but not enough not to betray him. But if Theseus is not your destiny, he is at least its starting point.

PHAEDRA: And did you really love him?

ARIADNE: A bit more than I thought. A bit less than I said.

PHAEDRA: Farewell, pure sister. Kiss me now, for we will probably not meet again until we meet in the land of Shadows, and there, we will have no lips for kisses. The wind is rising. I feel carried away by gusts that predict a storm. But, what's this, you are crying?

ARIADNE: It's nothing, Phaedra, just my last womanly sighs. After all, how can I deny you both this last pleasure, just when you are leaving. The only joy Theseus still expects from me is precisely my tears.

SCENE 9

A promontory in Naxos. Ariadne, then Bacchus (God).

ARIADNE: Solitude . . . I have known you in all your forms. The solitude of waiting, the solitude of love, the solitude of suffering and the regret of having suffered. Now, I drink you pure. The air is so transparent, I seem to breathe emptiness. Stable as the past, perfect as memory, the marble islet surges up from the fluid waters; the island rises so high that one can't tell if the surrounding waves are part of the sky or part of the sea. Silence, my lamentations will not soil you; as unyielding as yourself, my song of sad triumph will rise. But how cold it is, in spite of the sun. I will end up petrified in all this mineral beauty. My tears are congealing; my heartbeats, slowing down, grow faint. The blood flowing in my arteries must be now as blue as the deepest vein in the sky.

GOD: Ariadne, now it's my turn to make my entrance on stage.

ARIADNE: What, another visitor? Will I never have any peace?

GOD: I am Bacchus.

ARIADNE: Be on your way, Lord. I am not interested in tamed tigers, and all the wines in the world leave a bitter aftertaste.

GOD: What pride, Ariadne! I am the one you hoped to find in Theseus. Theseus was only a rough draft of me.

ARIADNE: I would have expected God to be more subtle. Right now, it's not a resemblance to Theseus that would attract me to a visitor.

GOD: Let's not speak badly of Theseus. He's the one who brought you to this island. You could not have made it here alone. And don't assume that look of distress, that classic pallor of the abandoned lover. You can't tell me you didn't force this poor man to leave.

ARIADNE: I did what I thought needed to be done. Besides, he would not have stayed.

GOD: His departure allowed you to meet God.

ARIADNE: You are nothing more than a one syllable word. You are only the shortest possible answer to all the questions of men.

GOD: Do you know a better one?

ARIADNE: Yes, the word "no" is just as short as the word God.

GOD: Hmm! You don't seem to realize, Ariadne, that I can make you immortal!

ARIADNE: I am already so. It's a privilege I share with every atom. Ariadne, sister of the fire, daughter of the air and rocks . . .

GOD: What I propose is conscious immortality.

ARIADNE: Thanks, I would just as soon sleep.

GOD: You are sleeping already. Your whole life was but a dream.

ARIADNE: One can't choose one's dreams . . . A grotesque father, an unclean mother, a monstrous brother, a lover not worthy of love, a sister condemned to crime. It should not surprise you that I would rather shut my eyes.

GOD: Among so many reasons for disgust, where does Ariadne fit in?

ARIADNE: That prude, that self-righteous woman who thought that only perfection was worthy of her? Ariadne also bores me. If I chose to live in this solitude, it was so that I would never be forced to hear her name.

GOD: Now that reassures me. I am beginning to think that you will not chase me from this rock as you did everyone else.

ARIADNE: The rock I chose was deserted, and you bring here a presence that is almost unbearable. The Being that you claim you are is thought by us to be invisible, and we have known for a long time that he does not speak. You talk. You have a form. I find you tiresomely human.

GOD: Look a little closer. Have you noticed how these little tufts of white hair on my breast form a star? And under my mane, as dark as ripe grapes, don't you see these little horns that show my kinship with the beasts in the fields and the crescents of the moon? And in my voice, can you only hear the seven note human scale? And this breath, Ariadne, deeper and warmer than that of any man?

ARIADNE: What, could you be? One and the same?

GOD: Not so fast. The question you are raising is so complicated that I sometimes can't figure it out myself.

ARIADNE: I understand, at least, that I don't understand. Maybe I was wrong to have urged Theseus to fight you.

GOD: One has to fight me before knowing me. That's where most of the victims are mistaken. They think that all they have to do is to die.

ARIADNE: Why did you keep Theseus waiting all night without giving him a chance to fight you then? You didn't deign show yourself. He crossed the threshold. The poor man behaved as well as he could. How can you be surprised that he didn't leave convinced?

GOD: Theseus saw Theseus. It's not the first time men have fashioned me after themselves. But don't give up on the salvation of your former lover. He will, perhaps, discover me some day in the guise of an old, blind man, or a boy dying in agony. As long as there is God, there is hope.

ARIADNE: But you have centuries on your side; your time is measured by almost endless cycles. Theseus, at best, has only about fifty more years ahead of him. And what if he gets lost in those corridors where every exit looks like the next? You ran the concession stand at the fair. You are responsible for all this claptrap. Will you guide him towards yourself? Will you grant him five minutes more when the game is over?

GOD: Don't butt in where you don't belong, Ariadne. Don't forget that etiquette forbids asking questions of gods and kings.

ARIADNE: Phaedra's destiny concerns me. Will she meet up with you?

GOD: Surely. I will devour her.

ARIADNE: How awful!

GOD: Not at all. Phaedra will find me handsome.

ARIADNE: So that I don't even have the privilege of a unique encounter. Any old road leads to you.

GOD: Does that bother you?

ARIADNE: No. But what about the fourteen victims? We abandoned them to their suffering as if they were unclaimed goods in a train depot. I am not interested in a happiness that millions of dead cannot share.

GOD: Another unsolvable problem! Don't turn down the sky as it opens for you, little creature. And yet it might not have opened had you not asked that question.

ARIADNE: I would rather not leave the island.

GOD: You don't have to. It has been rising imperceptibly. We are already floating.

ARIADNE: A constellation is also an island. But where were you hiding before Theseus left?

GOD: More or less everywhere. But I never show myself before the last ship has set sail.

ARIADNE: What is happening? This mane of yours has turned into myrtle, into lily of the valley? These swollen muscles are rocks with veins of sardonyx . . . How handsome you are, Rock of Ages. You are stretching; you are changing. From rock you turn into crystal, ice-floe, great white cloud. Neither man nor beast, perhaps not even God. Outside of names. Outside of kingdoms.

GOD: Press closer to my breast. You could fall from this height. Are you still cold?

ARIADNE: I am no longer crying. I am warm like an exhausted traveler who sinks into snow to sleep. My own voice hardly reaches me. The whiteness filling my eyes is as blinding as the darkest night. For the first time, I am aware that I am sleeping.

GOD: Sleep, my child. Rest your head on my chest. The heart of the whole world beats there.

ARIADNE: How simple it is! I never knew how sweet it is to give in. Now I am no longer afraid of dying.

GOD: You are already dead, Ariadne. And it is thus that your eternal life begins.

SCENE 10

On the ship anchored within sight of Athens. Theseus, Phaedra, Autolycos.

THESEUS: Look, Phaedra, straight across, on this hill, the point of Athena's helmet. From here, the statue looks tiny. It weighs at least twelve tons, and costs eight hundred staters. Here, close by, the smokestacks of Piraeus. To the right, the yacht club with its bathhouses on the beach, and its well heated swimming pool. We are going to enjoy together the pleasure of big city living.

PHAEDRA: Why are the bells tolling? And why are all the flags at half-mast? Why is the crowd dressed in black? Has the city been struck by a plague, or are they mourning someone?

THESEUS: My venerable father. The doctors warned me long ago. To be spared a few moments of anxiety, my father had requested that my ship would carry a white sail if I was safe and sound, and victorious. A fatal shock. My father who loved me . . . The pilot who just came on board brought me the sad news. Yet, I specifically cautioned Autolycos not to raise the black sails.

AUTOLYCOS: What! Would you repeat that, please?

THESEUS: Surely you can't deny that I had given you detailed instructions, myself, right here, a little while back when the Pleiades were setting? Besides, there will be no punishment whatsoever. Not the shadow of any official blame. Mistakes can happen, even on the best run ships.

AUTOLYCOS: Indeed, the most specific instructions. Sir, my shoulders are strong enough to carry the weight of the old man's death.

THESEUS: Alas, poor Aegeus! For me, Phaedra, the time of responsibilities has begun. How beautiful you will be on the morning of the coronation!

PHAEDRA: Theseus, I am very upset about this news. I had hoped to make my father-in-law love me.

THESEUS: We don't have much time. Reporters are gathering on the quay. Let's agree on a story that spares the families of the victims uselessly atrocious details of what happened. I intend to tell them that, after my victory over the Minotaur, the fourteen hostages chose to go inland and explore the country.

AUTOLYCOS: Unfortunately, your Majesty, there's already proof that your heroic undertakings did not purge the earth of one of its monsters. One of my dolphin friends ran into the Minotaur somewhere around here; he was disguised as a sea serpent. You will probably meet him somewhere on your road, or on that of your son.

THESEUS: Autolycos, for all the gold in the world . . .

AUTOLYCOS: That's too much and too vague. Why don't you offer me this ship, and I'll turn it into a fishing boat. Besides, you won't be going anywhere, anymore.

THESEUS: No, I won't be going away anymore. From now on, my royal duties will attach me to this shore. I intend to reorganize the government. The constitution of Crete gave me some good ideas. And it is about time that I find an experienced tutor for my son.

PHAEDRA: That's right, you have a son. How old is he?

THESEUS: He is twelve. He's a very wild child. I am not sure how he'll take to a step-mother.

PHAEDRA: Twelve? I hope, Theseus, that I will be able to make Hippolytus love me.

END

The Little Mermaid

A theatrical divertissement after the fairy tale by

Hans Christian Andersen

[1942]

Characters:

The Little Mermaid
The Water Witch
The Princess of Norway
The Prince of Denmark
The Count Ulrich
The Page Egon
The Dwarf Gog
The Dwarf Megog
A Chorus of Mermaids
A Chorus of Bird-Angels

PART ONE

At the Bottom of the Sea.

THE MERMAIDS: (*Singing, shaking their long hair.*) Ah, Ah, Ah, white, blue as waves. Ah, Oh, Hi, Gray as clouds and seagull wings! Ah, Ah, Black as the storms lashing at sails!

We are purple as the sea at sunset when the sun bleeds, pale as the light at noon when the fisherman, confused by so much transparency, wonders if he shouldn't cast his nets in the sky,—and, at night, we are what shadows are made of, the luminous dark, the green eyes of the abyss, and the damp long hair of the moon in the East.

On winter mornings, under a white sky, we leap like whales in the gray waves, a heavy sea herd and we jump, on summer days, like dolphins, on the rocks of Sicily. On stormy nights, in the open sea, far from sails, far from ropes, far from masts, far from all creakings or cries, far from the shores, from caves or reefs, far from all thunder echoing, our sharp voices erupt and sing, the only cry of the silent waves.

Swallowed up, dilating our divine gills, we prowl in submerged forests, like so many musing fish, spreading their pearly seeds in the cold womb of the sea. We rush like shark on the corpses of the drowned. Women of the abyss, eternal beasts, we speed along warm currents like amorous eels: opaline, swollen with dreams like jellyfish, we drift under the moon.

FIRST MERMAID: Where to?

SECOND MERMAID: Hunting with whales among green blocks of ice.

THIRD MERMAID: Where to?

FOURTH MERMAID: To gather coral twigs.

SECOND MERMAID: And you, where are you going?

FIFTH MERMAID: To a blond beach by a blue sea, where there are big tree trunks made of stone, the remains of a sunken city; trees white and smooth as human skin. I wrap my tail around them and rub my scales against the marble.

FIRST MERMAID: You, where are you going?

SIXTH MERMAID: To inspect the old ship, the big wooden hull bearded sailors called us from, stretching their hairy arms. I saw the battle: they are all dead; the prow is stuck in a sandbar. I slip, like a fish, in the gutted hull; I look for golden helmets among the shattered skulls.

THIRD MERMAID: Where do you go?

SEVENTH MERMAID: To sleep on rocks.

THIRD MERMAID: And you?

SECOND MERMAID: Leave her alone. She's the crazy mermaid. She puts human words into her songs. Come. Let's go.

FIFTH MERMAID: Faster. Let's get out of here. A shadow crawls on the bottom of the sea.

FIRST MERMAID: It's the Water Witch, the ugliest woman of the abyss, the beast with the shark teeth, with the lobster eyes, with the octopus arms, the eater of mermaid flesh. Quick!

SEVENTH MERMAID: Quick before her tentacles get in our hair!

(They run away. The Little Mermaid remains seated in the hollow of a rock, she holds in her lap the head of a statue; it is covered with seashells and seaweed.)

THE WATER WITCH: (Screaming.) Who are you, you who do not flee, and who strip me of the pleasure of making everything scatter before me in the calm waters. Aren't you afraid of the ugliest of creatures, of the eater of blue and white flesh?

(The Little Mermaid sighs.)

THE LITTLE MERMAID: Why should I fear you? I am being devoured by my own heart.

THE WATER WITCH: Your heart? Warm-blooded beast, little female whale, what use is your heart except to pump this viscous liquid flowing iridescent on the sea when a fisherman hits you with a harpoon. What is the matter with you?

THE LITTLE MERMAID: I'm in love.

THE WATER WITCH: (Frightened.) No, not that, you betray your kingdom. No love allowed at the ocean's depth.

THE LITTLE MERMAID: If I'm a traitor, I've been one for centuries, yes, centuries. I'm already using numbers like a human being. Once, when ships had red sails and three benches of men rowing, I ventured to this sea, bluer than all others, that sailors call the Aegean. A ship, disemboweled by a rock on the surface of the water, dropped its cargo—treasures we didn't know how to use appeared: broken jars spread their perfume on the sea. A white form sank to the bottom; first I thought it was the corpse of the most handsome of men. But I was wrong: he has been sleeping now for centuries, still uncorrupted, even though he has been lying on this underwater beach all this time. And every day, I cradle his heavy head on my knees. Look! I've even gotten used to these strange props they call legs. And every night, I go up to the surface very cautiously, and I look at the men on all the shores of the world. But until the other day, I had never seen one as handsome.

THE WATER WITCH: No, they are all ugly. Their best swimmers move like frogs.

THE LITTLE MERMAID: And, until the other day, I had never seen such a handsome man. But yesterday, a calm and moonless night, I ventured into a fjord. The lights of the royal castle were almost still on the dark, smooth waters. I was floating on my back, surrounded by a flight of curlews, ensnared by the sound of human music. Their voices are not as beautiful as ours but they own instruments we've never heard. And, suddenly on the terrace lit by torches, I saw the Prince. The night wind made his cape unfurl. His face was as beautiful as this one, and almost as white. Leaning on the railing, he was looking at the sea, dreamingly. And right away, I loved him.

THE WATER WITCH: You're not the first mermaid to want the son of a man. Didn't you show him your breasts? Didn't you sing?

(The Little Mermaid shudders.)

THE LITTLE MERMAID: No. I've seen drowned corpses with dead eyes, swollen bellies, stiff feet. I don't want to drag him into an element that's not his own, seduced, murdered by water voices.

THE WATER WITCH: Yet, they say that the flesh of a man one loves is particularly tasty. Alas, I'm not speaking through personal experience, not having the allurements of golden breasts or a silver voice.

THE LITTLE MERMAID: I love not only his flesh, but him, I love the whole man; I love him living. Everything about him fills me with a curiosity as avid as thirst or hunger. I want to inhale the air he breathes, to bite into the foods he tastes. (To think that before I would spit out those sour apples that, cast off from terrestrial gardens, would drift on the water!) I would like to look at the ocean from a distance, like him, like a stranger who doesn't know the secrets of the abyss. To walk like him, on that land where he places his feet.

THE WATER WITCH: Walk. That's blasphemy.

THE LITTLE MERMAID: (Lowering her head.) I know, but what can I do, oh, mother-of-all-terrors. If I drag my body on the pebbly beach, the king's washerwomen would beat me to death with their paddles the way they killed an old sick Triton warming himself in the sun the other day. Soldiers would jab at me with their lances for the pleasure of seeing my oily blood ooze out. Or a crafty fisherman would drag me through town and would show the Mermaid in a glass box for one of those coins men buy bread with. Oh, I wish I were nothing more than a woman, with nothing but womanly charms.

THE WATER WITCH: Every man is surrounded by hundreds of women he doesn't look at twice.

THE LITTLE MERMAID: At least they don't fill him with disgust, or surprise, or terror. Their chance at winning him, however slight, is a human chance. They don't drag in their wake the depth and its waves; their heart is their only abyss. I wish I had two white feet so that I could walk behind my prince on the roads at twilight, two solid bare feet. I yearn for human legs the way certain men are rumored to have yearned for wings.

THE WATER WITCH: You are committing the worst offense: you want to change elements, to change species. Are you really determined?

(The Little Mermaid gives a little cry of joy.)

THE LITTLE MERMAID: Do you know a way, Sister of Leviathan?
THE WATER WITCH: What will you give me for it?

(The Little Mermaid moves back, dropping the statue head.)

THE LITTLE MERMAID: I have nothing, Mother, Mermaids are naked. And these bracelets are common pearls you can gather in the corners of the sea.

THE WATER WITCH: And your voice? Don't you think that I'm tired of being an animal howling like a dog on a chain. (Have you heard them on the shore by the fishermen's huts in the long fall night?) Give me your voice and I'll give you those solid props that tremble and bend for prayer, for fear and for love.

(Crawling on the ground, the Little Mermaid moves back.)

THE LITTLE MERMAID: My voice!
THE WATER WITCH: (Wildly.) Let me suck your voice.
THE LITTLE MERMAID: Without my voice, how will I tell him that I love him?
THE WATER WITCH: (Cajolingly.) Won't you have your eyes? Won't you have your body? Won't you have your dancing? I'll give you feet gifted for dancing.
THE LITTLE MERMAID: Alas, scaly tail! Pivot of my body, spiral attaching me to

the sea. What will I become if you cut off half of me?

THE WATER WITCH: First, I'll scrape your tail with my stone knife. Then I'll slowly bring these mother-of-pearl scales to a boil in my caldron. And when the liquid will have boiled over three times, I'll throw it on your bleeding tail. You'll come out of this torture with two slim legs, with pure knees, with white feet, with toenails pink and gay as those of a newborn babe.

THE LITTLE MERMAID: White feet with pink toenails to walk with my Prince on those little perfumed seaweeds called flowers.

THE WATER WITCH: The land of men is very hard. You'll hurt with every step, with every movement; it will be as if beach stones were hitting you in the heart each time. But you'll have to smile, smile with that mouth that can no longer scream.

THE LITTLE MERMAID: In the presence of my Prince, I could no more not smile than water not reflect the sun to the sun. Come! My mind's made up. Eat my voice. Get your knife ready.

THE WATER WITCH: (*Rushing towards her.*) Your voice, your lips!

THE LITTLE MERMAID: No, wait a minute. Let me first sing, for my Prince, very softly, the song he will not hear. My death song. My last song:

> Love is a darker, colder chill
> Than the sea wind in the night air.
> Love has me now and love will kill.

> (Remember my song when I won't be there.)

> Like a rock in the sun alone,
> I let your light warm me at noon.
> The fire will blow up the stone.

> (Remember love; the heart is dust so soon.)

> Hold me against your heart to sleep
> Love is a pit dark clouds invade
> Seaweed I float, drift down the deep.

> (Remember Grief when you're like me, a shade.)

PART TWO

By the Sea.

The Prince is strolling on the beach accompanied by Count Ulrich, his aide-de-camp and followed by two dwarfs.

THE PRINCE: The truth is, my dwarfs, that you are happier than the Prince, your future is set; you will make the same faces and gestures your whole life long. (Don't cry Gog, you're handsome in your own way.) As for me, my youth is over; my freedom has folded its wings. My shoulders are encumbered by royalty and the pompous cares of State. The ship is being rigged out, the presents are stacked up in the hold; tomorrow the Prince of Denmark will sail to his cold Norwegian Betrothed. Farewell, city charmers, faces caught by the light of a red lantern. And you, fishermen's daughters, little gray shrimp at the edge of a pool. And you, Gypsies, met at the bend of a road, reading the future. Farewell elusive dream woman made of froth and desire. Ulrich, my friend, you won't recognize me disguised as a husband and king.

COUNT ULRICH: May I remind the Prince that he does not know the heiress of the kingdom of Norway. His Majesty has not yet set eyes on his fiancee.

THE PRINCE: So what! A doll probably, a dummy in a white ermine coat. Alas, a queen is part of a king's trappings.

COUNT ULRICH: The Prince forgets too quickly that his lot is worthy of envy. Many men would give their lives for one hour of royalty.

THE PRINCE: And me, I would give my whole royal existence for one hour like this one, a simple stroll along the beach. My wild adventures were but the banners and noisy fanfare of my freedom; it's that very freedom I'll miss and the carefree existence of a man sleeping at the crossroads of the future. Look: a fisherman pulls in his net. It caught no other treasure than a few flakes of foam; a white bird is gliding, buffeted by the wind; the sand absorbs each wet ring imprinted by the waves. And the slightest puddle left by high tide is a mirror for mermaids.

COUNT ULRICH: His highness is a poet. I don't know which is more admirable, the realism of his images or his gift for refreshing the most used metaphors.

THE PRINCE: How many nights did I spend on this beach trying to put the magic sounds of the sea into words! But poets are seldom eye-witnesses to miracles, and this shore where any old woman thinks she'll meet Neptune, and where mermaids are supposed to sing, furnishes the Prince only with fish for his supper on Holy Friday.

COUNT ULRICH: Old wives tales! Superstitious nonsense. The education of the masses, My Lord, will be one of the tasks of your reign.

(The dwarf Gog whispers mysteriously, a finger against his thick lips.)

GOG: Not so fast Uncle Ulrich! I'm somewhat of an expert when it comes to music. And last night, from that dog house by the sea in which I live, I heard something like a woman's voice howling at the moon. Not a sob, but a song so sweet it made me want to die. A shudder ran all over my hump. (I'm somewhat of an expert in witchcraft, having been born on the island of Rugen.) I got up.

COUNT ULRICH: So what? Probably some chambermaid, some washerwoman giving birth.

GOG: (*Humbly.*) No! Even though a real live washerwoman would be fairer game for a dwarf than a dreamed-of mermaid. But the terrace was deserted. Except for a sentinel snoring at his post. (Begging your pardon.) And the water sprite dove back into the sea before these little legs of mine could reach her.

COUNT ULRICH: Too bad. I would have given a pretty penny to witness the coupling of a fish and an ugly dwarf. The lash, the lash, My Lord, for dwarfs who lie, or the iron collar for dwarfs who drink.

THE PRINCE: Quiet! What right do I have to refuse the universe the possibility of a mermaid? Better discuss the Spanish wine imported for the wedding supper. But what have we here? Egon, my page, is coming towards us dragging behind him something that is struggling on the sand.

EGON: (*Out of breath.*) A woman, your highness, a woman. I found an unconscious woman behind this rock, half lying in water. Look, I am parting her hair. She doesn't bite; she seems very gentle.

THE PRINCE: (*Leaning over her.*) No, I don't know her. Strange that such beauty should have escaped the Prince's notice.

MEGOG: Speak of mermaids and here they are. (*He lifts her dress.*) The tail. No, she has legs, and beautiful legs at that!

THE PRINCE: That's enough. She has beautiful light eyes. She's probably some virtuous child, a merchant's daughter who ran away from home because of a family quarrel. Young Lady!

EGON: She doesn't understand Danish. I tried.

THE PRINCE: Do you understand me, young lady? (*The Little Mermaid nods.*) Can you answer me? (*The Little Mermaid shakes her head and cries.*) No more voice than tail, my good dwarfs. The mermaid vanishes and what we have left is a weeping child. Tell me, did you run away from home? (*The Little Mermaid nods.*) I thought so. Did you commit one of those maidenly offenses? (*The Little Mermaid shakes her head.*) What, no crime, my virtuous child? Are you in love with someone? (*The Little Mermaid bursts into tears.*) He cheats on you or he ignores you? Dry your tears, my child. The best of men would just as soon sleep with a slut as with the prettiest of Angels. We'll have to find this child's parents, Count Ulrich.

EGON: Look, My Lord. This green silk dress was woven on Oriental looms. These feet have never walked on beach pebbles nor on city pavement. And this pearl bracelet would pay a queen's ransom.

THE PRINCE: Good God! You're right, my page. She must be some nobleman's daughter kidnapped by pirates and mourned, perhaps, by an entire populace in some distant land. Answer, young lady, do you know how to write? Can you draw your name on the sand? (*The Little Mermaid shakes her head.*) Are you a king's daughter? (*The Little Mermaid nods.*)

COUNT ULRICH: That's what they all say. My Lord, I bet she's a trollop, a slut brought here at great expense by the procuress of the Golden Boot Inn. Most likely, she was lost along the way following some handsome boy.

THE PRINCE: Slut or queen, her eyes are so big you could drown in them. What do you think, Gog?

GOG: Phew! A fisherman's daughter who stole her jewels from some Madonna statue. She smells of the tide.

MEGOG: Give her to us, Highness. She'll have to earn a living like everyone else. I'll teach her to make faces.

THE PRINCE: Hands off, jealous dwarfs. Are you afraid of the unfair competition of Beauty? But really, what will happen to you if you can't tell us your name or country. Do you know how to spin wool or silk? Can you prepare exotic confections, brew magical potions, or heal the sick with herbs? (*The Little Mermaid shakes her head.*)

COUNT ULRICH: I bet she knows how to make love, My Lord.

THE PRINCE: Do you know how to make love, young lady? Can you make your body vibrate like a harp or like a gong? Or wrap it around a man's body like a scarf? (*The Little Mermaid crawls to his feet and kisses his hands.*) What passion! How you tempt me! My new resolutions are only a half hour old. But what good is a lover who's mute and wouldn't be able to say my name tenderly? God did not grant you a voice. (*The Little Mermaid weeps.*)

MEGOG: My grandfather used to say that the best match was between a blind man and a mute woman.

THE PRINCE: Don't cry, my child. Most people talk just to talk and almost all are deaf and blind. True, nothing equals a pure voice to cure our suffering or to lift us to heaven, but there are certain poses that are worth all songs, certain gestures more precious than music. Do you know how to dance? (*The Little Mermaid rises, painfully tries a few dance steps, then crumbles on the ground with a moan.*) What? Hold her up, Egon! She is dying!

COUNT ULRICH: She's probably a madwoman, an epileptic. Don't touch her, My Lord.

THE PRINCE: (*Kneeling.*) No, No, all the charm in the world was in her gestures, and the movement of her clumsy little feet evoked the oblique flight of a tern. Look! I've never held such small feet. But how she is shaking, and we'll never know whether it's from fear, from cold or from rapture. The poor child is probably dying of hunger. Egon, take her on board; and have a good meal prepared for her. And don't forget to have matron inspect her long hair; we don't want any vermin on the boat. Gentlemen, the voyage will be long, and at night, on the decks drenched by the fogs of the open sea, her dancing will distract us. Do you hear, young lady? And who knows? Maybe one night, even though you won't be able to answer, I'll feel like whispering some sweet words of love in your ear. Are you happy?

Go, go. And as for us, my friends, let's not forget to ask, each time we stop somewhere, if pirates haven't kidnapped some local beauty. Policing the seas is the constant headache of kings.

PART THREE

On the Prince's Boat
Anchored off the Coast of Norway.

The two dwarfs are sitting on a stepladder by the entrance of the royal tent.

GOG: Damn trip!

MEGOG: Damn country!

GOG: But yesterday, the wedding supper was excellent! (*Burps.*) The King of Norway's cook knows how to do things right.

MEGOG: The King of Norway's cook be damned! I was sitting next to the stove and he chased me away with his red hot spatula.

GOG: You don't know how to go about it! The scullery maid saved all the turkey bones for me. (*He whispers in his ear.*)

MEGOG: Ah, Ah, Ah. You old bastard, you!

GOG: On top of it all, we'll have to make up new tricks for Norwegian tastes. And the Princess, what do you think of her? (*The Dwarf Megog whispers in his ear.*) Ah, Ah. As for me, I fancy the little mute one better.

MEGOG: You didn't have any luck with her, did you? Do you remember the day she bit you?

GOG: Ouch! Teeth like a shark.

MEGOG: I think she's disgusting. Everyone raved about her during the trip. (*Gog rubs his shoulders.*)

GOG: She wasn't even whipped once!

MEGOG: Pretty eyes don't get whipped.

GOG: Fish eyes! A stinking idiot. I can't get over the idea that there is some magic involved here.

MEGOG: I'll speak to the bishop about it as soon as we get back to Copenhagen. What a nice fire she'll make. (*They laugh.*)

GOG: If you ask me you'd be better off denouncing her to the future queen.

(*They laugh harder.*)

MEGOG: I'm fed up by now. It makes me sick to sit next to her at dinner and see her gobbling up raw fish. The best thing would be to throw her back in the water.

GOG: Excellent idea my Hercules! You take her by the head.

MEGOG: And you by the feet, my Samson! Hoop la!

(*They guffaw with laughter. The Prince, in court costume, makes his entrance. He is followed by Count Ulrich and the Little Mermaid. She is wearing leotards.*)

THE PRINCE: Ulrich, take care of the musicians. Did you teach them the new madrigal by Roland de Lassus? Let everything be ready; have them standing with their instruments tucked under their chin. And, as soon as my royal beloved sets foot on this ship, let the music swell, wave, furl and unfurl like a banner: Ah, at the very touch of those sweet little velvet clad feet, the whole ship will shudder with love, like a cello. Ulrich!

COUNT ULRICH: Prince.

THE PRINCE: You were next to me during the procession in church, in the palace. You saw the princess. Ah, Ulrich, don't tell me she is beautiful unless you have a new word meaning beauty, fresh as dawn, invented for her alone.

COUNT ULRICH: Highness, the Princess is worthy of the Prince. The Prince is worthy of the Princess.

THE PRINCE: Go, Count Ulrich! Go take care of the musicians! (*Count Ulrich leaves. The Prince turns to the Little Mermaid.*) And you, my child, do you know the dance I taught you? I'm counting on you to express my happiness in delightful gestures. Are you ready? (*The Little Mermaid nods.*) Child, lift your eyes toward me. Look at me as though you understood. Perhaps God created you so that I could confide my secret to a mute. Child who sweetened the sea's loneliness for me, I don't thank you for your body nor for your dancing (all beautiful women have bodies and some of them know how to dance). I thank you for your silence which allows me to speak without being interrupted, approved or contradicted. I'm in love, my child. My young man's wisdom, so like the wisdom of old age, has fallen from my shoulders like a winter coat. I thought I was seeking a queen, out of duty, and for the first time I understand why men placed the image of a woman clasping an infant to her bosom in their churches. For the first time I understand the happiness of the milkboy walking at night with the milkmaid; and that love is a mystery and not just a sad pleasure, and that each kiss given by perishable lips is stronger than death. Yesterday in church, when she turned towards me to say "I do," the words were like a perfect golden circle. I realized, for the first time, that life is not just a multi-colored rag shred by the North Wind, a Carnival costume one masquerades in to drink and dance, but a solid piece

of cloth our children will still be able to use. And at evening, after the ban-
quet, when she stepped on the balcony to sing . . . but alas, poor little
voiceless girl, how will you ever know what heights a woman's song can
reach? (*The Little Mermaid covers her face with her hands.*) Listen, little one.
Don't be sad. My life is going to change but you will be as well treated as my
falcons after the hunting season, or my jugglers after the Christmas
holidays. If you'd like, in Copenhagen, I'll entrust you to the Abbess of the
Convent of the Crown of Thorns. You'll be happy in their beautiful walled-
in garden, like a flower reserved for God. (*The Little Mermaid shakes her head.
The Prince smiles.*) What, no convent, little wild plant? Would you prefer
Dame Balbine's house, The Golden Boot? The girls there are fed gourmet
dishes and dressed in gowns brought from Paris by the same couriers as
those who bring in gowns for the queen. In the old days, I myself would
spend my evenings there, from time to time. (*The Little Mermaid shakes her
head.*) You're being very difficult, my child. Well, we'll find something, don't
worry. Ah, and be sure not to forget that dance step where you hang upside
down like a little seal in a graceful, slightly comic manner. Ah, the violins.
(*Music.*) Quiet, my heart. A whole world of joy draws near on two little fur
slippers. My queen! (*He kneels.*)

(*The Princess enters followed by her ladies-in-waiting and escorted by Count Ulrich.*)

THE PRINCE: My queen! For you are my queen even more than my soul. My
soul. For you my soul even more than my heart. I thought I came to you
loaded with treasures and experience, but the child drops the pebbles,
picked up off the road, so that he can receive the perfect pearl. I thought I
brought you my passions, but you are the one who brings me this love fresh
as the beginning of the world, pure as the evening and the morning star! I
feel naive as a child, tongue-tied as a schoolboy, empty-handed as a slave,
perhaps because on this day, I accede to my dignity as a man and as a king. I
thought I was bringing you my melancholy but I cast off these worn rags,
and I wrap myself in your joy as in a golden cloth. I thought I brought you
my crown but what can I bring a swan, only water and sky? I wish I were a
tramp at your feet, a beggar at your door so that I would owe you my bread
as I owe you my heart.

THE PRINCESS: What are you saying? I prefer you king.

COUNT ULRICH: The Princess is right.

(*The maids of honor leave, curtsying.*)

THE PRINCE: Sit down, Princess, on this fur-covered couch. This boat is small
like a floating nest. Like halcyons of Ancient Greece, we'll drift tonight on a
calm sea, a sea favorable to our nuptials.

THE PRINCESS: I was warned that you were very learned. You speak like those books of poetry with which they taught me to read. No, this crossing at your side will not be long, and soon Copenhagen's pleasures will make us forget the ocean's monotony.

THE PRINCE: The evening wind won't bother you. I had drapes hung around the tent.

THE PRINCESS: Good. The sight of waves makes me seasick.

THE PRINCE: That doesn't surprise me. This insipid spectacle grates on the nerves and plunges the mind into a kind of lethargy. What could be more boring than these curves, all alike, this black following the blue which is in turn followed by blue-gray. But even on this ship we have our distractions; we have musicians, jugglers, and here are dwarfs who learned new tricks just for you.

(*The dwarfs bow and make faces. Grotesque music. The Princess bursts out laughing.*)

THE PRINCESS: Oh, oh. How funny he is. And the other one with his mouth split to his ears!

THE PRINCE: Ah, her laughter sparkles like a spring waterfall. Good dwarfs, you'll each get a gold coin.

(*The dwarfs bow and leave.*)

THE PRINCE: (*Introducing the Little Mermaid.*) And this one is an abandoned child, a little mute whose dancing helped while away the time during the trip.

(*The Little Mermaid shyly executes a dance step while the music plays something sad and complicated.*)

THE PRINCESS: I don't like her. She dances badly. She has ugly eyes.

THE PRINCE: (*To the Little Mermaid.*) Enough, stop. Go!

(*The Little Mermaid leaves.*)

THE PRINCE: It doesn't matter, Princess; we'll put her on shore at the very first stop.

THE PRINCESS: I don't like her. Why do we need dancing girls, Prince? I myself will teach you Norwegian dances.

THE PRINCE: How delightful! Music! (*He signals for music.*)

THE PRINCESS: No, Prince, not tonight. Remember that I just left my good father. (*She pulls out a handkerchief.*)

THE PRINCE: My beloved, don't regret your childhood. I promise to give you another, better one, richer, more to your liking as a woman. We'll go hunting on estuaries for teal and wild duck, our horses will trample fields of primroses underfoot. In wintertime, we'll leave tracks side by side, in the snow, fast Angels unfurling the wings of our coats behind us. Oh, all these places I used to haunt aimlessly, now I'll see them again, led by a celestial guide like Tobias by his Seraphim! And when we are old, beloved, sitting by the royal fireplace, we'll look back on our days, one by one, like a set of precious stones. And when I lie dying, having left behind me sons more handsome than me and daughters who resemble you, you will clasp me in your lovely white arms; death, with you by my side, will only be a short sleep until the Dawn of Resurrection. But what's this, my beloved yawns? (*The Princess falls asleep.*) The day has been long and tiring for my Princess. And my silly chatter was not useless since it put her to sleep. Go, Count Ulrich, have the sweetest of lullabies played very softly. Sleep in peace, my gentleness. I will lie down beside you to dream of you, and later, when auspicious stars appear in the Orient, the ship's astrologer will signal the start of our wedding. (*He falls asleep.*)

(*The mizzen sail, which was the backdrop for the scene and which hangs like a curtain in an alcove, is removed. Very soft music. Until the end of the play, the boat will be rocked by a slow, cradle-like movement. Holding a knife, the Little Mermaid reappears on the deserted deck. Her pantomime expresses rancor, hatred, hesitation and suffering. The Prince moves in his sleep and puts his arm under the Princess' neck.*)

THE PRINCE: My joy. My soul.

(*The Little Mermaid takes a step forward. Suddenly the sound of the sea swells becomes the voices of the mermaids.*)

THE MERMAIDS: Kill, kill, kill. Kill this man whose heart is made of stone and this woman whose heart is made of plaster. Sink your knife into their horrible lungs that serve as gills. You have nothing in common with this earthworm race. He betrayed you. Revenge yourself. He did worse than betray you, he slighted you, take revenge. He did worse than slight you, he did not recognize you, take revenge. Come back to us, little sister, come back to us, pearl of the sea.
Deprived of you, the Ocean laments and the salmon are sad, and the coral less pink. Give up those awkward legs, absurd terrestial tools, useless to mermaids who ride the waves. Kill! Kill! Kill! Let that lukewarm juice they call their blood flow on your absurd feet. And the spell will be broken: scales will cover your thighs, and fins will grow out of those heels! You will find your shining tail again, undulating in the sea. Quick! The magic hour is almost here! Sirius throbs on the horizon. Kill! Wash the dirty blood of their hearts

off your feet. Crawl, drag your viscous tail on the deck. Throw yourself overboard into the sea that would drown the woman, but will joyfully press to her green bosom her Little Mermaid coming back. Come, help us push this ship on a reef, this ship that brought you pain will be wrecked and become nothing more than a toy for Triton children.

Come. You will regain your beautiful voice, your singing that seduces, your singing that kills. From now on, our immortal lives will be spent setting traps for mariners, these monsters who kill the creatures of the abyss. We'll drag them downward, by their feet, towards the deep. Sister of seals, of flying fish, of polar whales, kill, kill, kill, avenge the honor of the waves!

(The Little Mermaid takes a step forward. Suddenly, higher than the sails, the riggings, the masts, drowning out the Mermaids' voices, the sharp song of Bird-Angels is heard rising towards the sky.)

BIRD-ANGELS: Come, come, come. Forget, forget, forget. Forget these weighty creatures, these wingless flesh machines. Cast off these narrow lungs inhaling only a tiny part of the sky. Once for love, you gave up the substance of the green abyss, the viscous body of the depth, give up your earthly form now, reject the woman held captive by a deck, held down by gravity.

Come, come, come. Throw yourself into the water. Your soul will rise to us like a free seagull grazing the waves. Too pure for death, too high for love, winged cry, eternal heart, fly with us beyond the foam, beyond space. In the storm. In the sunlight. Come! Come! Come! Let go and come with us! Forget! Come! Come! Come!

(The Little Mermaid drops her knife. She stretches out her arms and is surrounded by the Bird-Angels.)

END

PAJ PLAYSCRIPT SERIES